One Year to a Successful Massage Therapy Practice

One Year to a Successful Massage Therapy Practice

Laura Allen, NCTMB

Wolters Kluwer Health | Lippincott Williams & Wilkins

Philadelphia • Baltimore • New York • London
Buenos Aires • Hong Kong • Sydney • Tokyo

Acquisitions Editor: John Goucher
Managing Editor: Jennifer Walsh
Marketing Manager: Nancy Bradshaw
Production Editor: Kevin P. Johnson
Designer: Teresa Mallon
Compositor: International Typesetting and Composition

351 West Camden Street
Baltimore, MD 21201

530 Walnut Street
Philadelphia, PA 19106

9 8 7 6 5 4 3 2 1

Library of Congress Cataloging-in-Publication Data

Allen, Laura, NCTMB.
One year to a successful massage therapy practice / Laura Allen.
p. ; cm.
Includes bibliographical references and index.
ISBN-13: 978-0-7817-7120-7
ISBN-10: 0-7817-7120-X
1. Massage therapy—Practice. 2. Massage therapy—Marketing. I. Title.
[DNLM: 1. Massage—methods. 2. Marketing of Health Services—methods.
3. Practice Management, Medical. WB 537 A427o 2008]
RM722.A42 2008
615.8'22068—dc22

2007042280

DISCLAIMER

Care has been taken to confirm the accuracy of the information present and to describe generally accepted practices. However, the authors, editors, and publisher are not responsible for errors or omissions or for any consequences from application of the information in this book and make no warranty, expressed or implied, with respect to the currency, completeness, or accuracy of the contents of the publication. Application of this information in a particular situation remains the professional responsibility of the practitioner; the clinical treatments described and recommended may not be considered absolute and universal recommendations.

The authors, editors, and publisher have exerted every effort to ensure that drug selection and dosage set forth in this text are in accordance with the current recommendations and practice at the time of publication. However, in view of ongoing research, changes in government regulations, and the constant flow of information relating to drug therapy and drug reactions, the reader is urged to check the package insert for each drug for any change in indications and dosage and for added warnings and precautions. This is particularly important when the recommended agent is a new or infrequently employed drug.

Some drugs and medical devices presented in this publication have Food and Drug Administration (FDA) clearance for limited use in restricted research settings. It is the responsibility of the health care provider to ascertain the FDA status of each drug or device planned for use in their clinical practice.

To purchase additional copies of this book, call our customer service department at **(800) 638-3030** or fax orders to **(301) 223-2320.** International customers should call **(301) 223-2300.**

Visit Lippincott Williams & Wilkins on the Internet: http://www.lww.com. Lippincott Williams & Wilkins customer service representatives are available from 8:30 am to 6:00 pm, EST.

Dedicated to Champ
My friend, my husband, my rock
and to the memory of Norris,
I miss you every day.

ABOUT THE AUTHOR

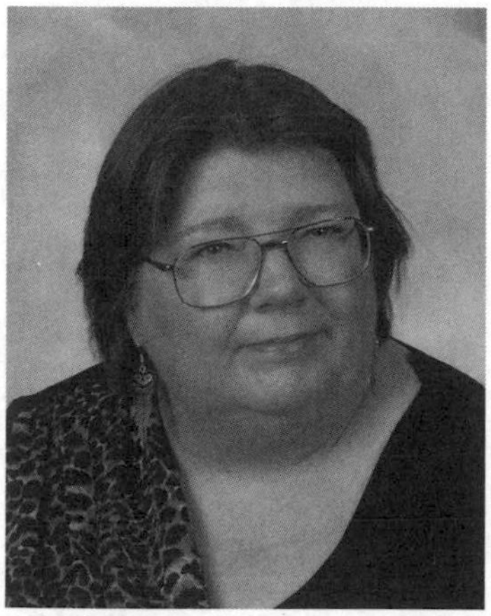

Laura Allen is a nationally certified massage therapist and bodyworker, and an approved provider of continuing education under the NCBTMB. She currently offers continuing education classes in Aromatherapy, Marketing, Professional Ethics, all levels of Reiki, Spa Techniques, and Structural Rebalancing. She has previously authored the *Plain & Simple Guide to Therapeutic Massage & Bodywork Certification* (Lippincott Williams & Wilkins, 2005), and currently teaches her popular class in How to Pass the NCE in massage schools and career colleges throughout North and South Carolina. She is on the visiting faculty at a number of schools, including the Obus School of Healing Therapies in Dublin, Ireland.

Laura acts as a private consultant to massage schools and educators as well as mentoring students from several different schools. She is active in the North Carolina Chapter of AMTA and the Carolina Emergency Response Massage Team that provides massage to emergency responders at disaster sites on a volunteer basis. She is currently serving a term as a therapist member on the North Carolina Board of Massage & Bodywork Therapy.

After more than twenty years as a busy restaurant owner and chef, Laura began practicing Healing Touch in 1993, and graduated from The Whole You School of Massage & Bodywork in Rutherfordton in 2000, where she served as an instructor and the school's administrator for five years. Laura also pursued an education in psychology with the intent of becoming a counselor, before deciding that her true path was relieving emotional stress and pain through bodywork. She enjoys doing research and is a past recipient of the North Carolina AMTA Community Service grant for her work with people in persistent vegetative states and other brain injuries. She is currently doing research on the efficacy of massage, aromatherapy, and other healing modalities on people who suffer from Tourette syndrome.

Laura is regionally well-known as a musician and songwriter in the mountains of western North Carolina and has made numerous public appearances over the last thirty years, including being featured on public radio, public television, and several recordings. She has been a member of the band Hogwild for over two decades and enjoys playing the guitar, piano, and harmonica professionally as well as for stress relief. She also enjoys creative writing and studying the Irish language, history, and culture.

She and her husband Champ, a builder by trade and a Reiki Master practitioner and teacher, are the owners of THERA-SSAGE, a clinic and educational facility staffed with over a dozen practitioners of different disciplines of bodywork, acupuncture, natural healing, and aesthetics. In addition to the classes they personally offer, they annually host a number of other massage and bodywork educators, as well as offering ongoing classes to the community in yoga, belly dancing, and other classes. Laura and Champ reside in Rutherfordton, North Carolina with their spoiled Chow, Smokey Bear.

PREFACE

Attending massage school was the beginning of one of the most exciting journeys I have ever undertaken. People who choose massage as a career are often walking their own path of self-discovery and self-healing. As a group, I think we're looking for more than just financial rewards; we get a sense of personal satisfaction in seeing the positive changes that take place in our clients as a result of our work. It's a dream come true when we can help others and make a great living at the same time.

If you are still in massage school, or a recent graduate, you can use this book as a tool to help you establish yourself as a massage therapist and build a successful practice, no matter what circumstances you're working in or intending to work in. If you are already a business and massage veteran, you can revitalize a practice that may have become stagnant or boring by following the suggestions in this book. I don't want to call this book a how-to manual, though some would. Instead, I would like for you to think of it as your roadmap to success. What do you do with a map when you're in a strange place? Right—you read it and you use it for guidance. Otherwise, the map's just a piece of paper with a nice drawing on it. Getting to your destination requires that you follow the directions on the map—by taking *action.*

Not all of the ideas in this book will apply to everyone's individual situation—but most will apply to most people's situations. Although this book is written by a massage therapist, primarily for massage therapists or massage therapy students, much of the marketing advice could easily be utilized by others in the complementary and alternative healing arts, such as chiropractors, acupuncturists, and naturopaths.

The Small Business Administration, on the web at **www.sba.gov,** gives a wonderful piece of advice: *"Never let a day pass without engaging in at least one marketing activity."* I've taken that concept to heart and it has worked for me. It will work for you as well. Of course, I can't guarantee that you'll be making a certain income a year after reading the book, but I feel confident that if you follow these suggestions, you'll be well on your way to having the practice you want.

Organization of This Book

The introduction to this book, *The Road to Success,* explains some of the traditional concepts of marketing. Part I, *Mapping Out Your Journey,* is the real beginning of your work—mapping out your road to success by defining your goals, developing a marketing budget and calendar that can co-exist in prosperous harmony, and avoiding common pitfalls. Part II, *Preparing for Your Trip,* is about getting yourself ready for prosperity by being sure all the basics are covered—things like choosing just the right name for your business, making a great presentation, getting informative and appealing business literature, and using your telephone as a sales tool in the best possible way. Part III, *The Path to Promotion,* addresses promoting your business by utilizing everything from methods that won't cost you a cent to advertising that will cost you as much money as you may want or have to spend, and how to make the best use of your hard-earned dollars by choosing your advertising venues wisely. Part IV, *Trip Tips,* is a resource guide in the form of appendices (massage therapy boards, national professional associations, sources for marketing materials, Internet resources, and a marketing calendar) to help you along on your trek to success.

As you read through the book, you'll see that each week has an activity for you to pursue. You don't need to do them in order, or even limit yourself to reading the chapters in order. I do recommend reading Parts I and II first, but thereafter, you will probably want to thumb through the chapters and find something you can fit into the week you're in. For instance, some of the activities may be built around holidays—and you may not be reading that chapter during holiday season. Feel free to read the chapters and do the journaling in any order you please, but the point is to do *something* to promote yourself every week for a year. I recommend that you record the date when you first applied the suggestion to your practice, and revisit the issue a year later and record what has happened in the interim as a result.

Features

The following features appear in most chapters to help you along your road to success.

My Personal Journey

This journal feature, which is the most important feature in the book, will encourage readers to try the techniques found in the chapter. The premise of this book is that the therapist has to be proactive in order to be successful; the journaling will keep them on task, both in taking action and in tracking their progress. Each journal page includes the following parts:

- **"This Week's Activity":** a concrete activity for the reader to perform, based on the chapter content—taking positive action in order to create prosperity.
- **"My Goals":** provides space for readers to identify their goals based on the chapter content and the activity.
- **"What's in my way?":** encourages readers to explore the obstacles facing them so that they can determine if the particular activity will or will not work for them. The true exploration is in whether or not there are real obstacles, or whether the perceived obstacles are just mental blocks of their own making.
- **"What action can I take to remedy the situation?":** encourages readers to move past the obstacles, real or perceived, by deciding on a positive course of action and then taking it.
- **"One Year Progress Update":** provides space for readers to return to each activity in a year to let them see how each activity did or did not work for them. It allows them to refine their marketing plan for the future.

Use the journal space as a place to think things through. For example, if you run across a suggestion in the book that you don't think will work, don't automatically discard it because you think it won't fit your particular case. Instead, write down four or five reasons why you think it won't work. If they're valid reasons, fine—but some of those times, you might see that it is your own laziness, pre-conditioning or negative attitude that is keeping you from trying new things. And that's the purpose of the exercise: to make yourself aware of self-sabotage. Don't feel compelled to just stick to my suggestions for success, either. If you hear of a marketing idea you'd like to try from another source, or come up with a great idea of your own, use the journal feature in the same way.

My Story

This feature contains personal anecdotes from former students and colleagues who have been generous enough to share their personal experiences about their quest for success. Each story explains how following the author's advice helped their massage practice.

Cautions

The highway has caution signs. They're not meant to make you give up on where you're going; they're meant for you to watch for a hazard that might get in your way. The same with the caution signs in this book. They're not meant to discourage you from marketing yourself and your business; they're meant to warn you of some of the possible pitfalls you might encounter along the way so you can avoid them.

Other Features

Throughout the book, there are road signs to guide you and cartoons to help you have a good time while traveling your course. This book doesn't contain learning objectives, because the only objective is for you to cultivate a successful massage practice, regardless of the situation you're in now. There also aren't any tests. The test is in whether or not you have the desire and the discipline to put these suggestions into action.

Additional Resources

One Year to a Successful Massage Therapy Practice includes additional resources for both instructors and students that are available on the book's companion website at thePoint.lww.com/Allen1year. Resources are also available via an Instructor's Resource CD-ROM.

Instructors

Approved adopting instructors will be given access to the following additional resources:

- Handouts, including a sample intake form, payment plan agreement, and business plan
- Lesson Plans
- PowerPoint presentations
- Templates of a tri-fold brochure and a sample business card

Students

Students who have purchased *One Year to a Successful Massage Therapy Practice* have access to the following resources:

- Handouts
- Templates

Organizing Yourself

Just as this book is organized, *you* are going to need some organization. Get out a brand-new file folder and label it "One Year to a Successful Massage Practice." Save your old marketing files, if you have any, and you can revisit them later and cull them for still-viable ideas. You may want to include a profit and loss sheet in the folder as well, so you can compare your financial situation today to your situation a year from now and see how things have changed for the better.

Bon Voyage!

The dictionary tells us that a journey is a "defined course of travel," *defined* being the key word. Using this book as a road map, taking real action, and journaling your activities will help you define and refine your goals as you head for prosperity. Confucius said, "A journey of a thousand miles begins with a single step." Resolve now to view each new day as an opportunity to grow personally, to grow your business, and to keep taking those steps on your journey to prosperity and personal enrichment. Good luck, and bon voyage!

Laura Allen, NCTMB
THERA-SSAGE
431 S. Main St., Ste. 2
Rutherfordton, NC 28139
828-288-3727
therassage@bellsouth.net
www.thera-ssage.com

REVIEWERS

Patty Berak
Director of Massage Therapy
Baker College of Clinton Township
Center Line, MI

Cindi Gill
Owner/Instructor
Body Business School of Massage Therapy
Durant, OK

Sam Gill
Owner/Instructor
Body Business School of Massage Therapy
Durant, OK

Janene Jaynes, LMT
Provo College
Provo, UT

Stacey Long
Assistant Director
Miami-Jacobs Career College
Dayton, OH

Nancy Smeeth, LMT
Connecticut Center for Massage Therapy
Wethersfield, CT

Robert Troy, LCMT
Dubuque, IA

ACKNOWLEDGMENTS

There are so many people who deserve thanks for their help on this book. First is my husband Champ, who is very gracious about my ignoring him for many hours at a time when I am writing. He has unquestioningly supported my every dream and desire since the day we met. Thanks to my mother, Margaret Lawson, who has cleaned my house and brought me food while I was too wrapped up in working to think about either. Thank you so much to the more than forty former students, teachers, and colleagues of mine who shared their experiences and wisdom for inclusion in the book. A big thank you to my staff members at THERA-SSAGE; they are the people who make our business continue to grow and prosper, and I am merely the ringleader. We laugh at work every day and I am grateful for that. Thank you to Cheryl Shew and everyone at The Whole You School of Massage & Bodywork for the education I received there and their ongoing support of my success. Thank you to my friends in the Sunday Night Music Club, who provide my stress relief and keep me sane. Thank you to John Goucher and the entire massage team at Lippincott Williams & Wilkins, who treat you like family and nurture your book like a growing baby; it is impossible to imagine a group of people any more wonderful to work with than they are. Thank you also to the reviewers, who take it and make it much better. I am truly blessed.

CONTENTS

Introduction: The Road to Success

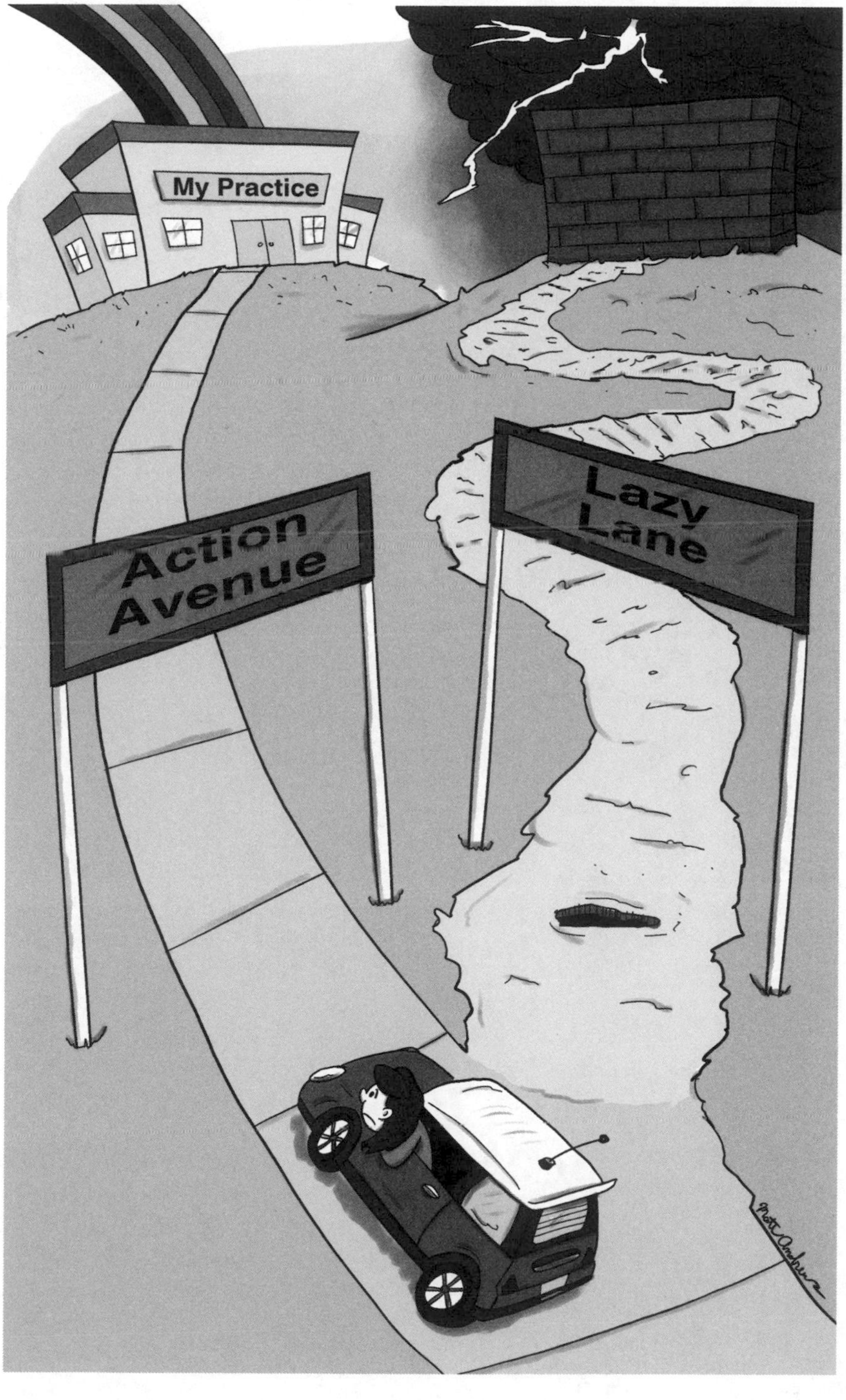

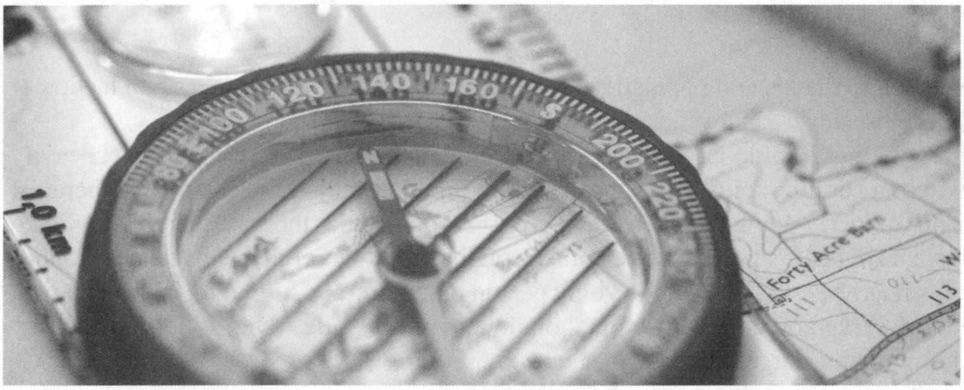

There is a road to success, and this book is going to be your road map. For the next year, think of yourself as a traveler along that road, and think of marketing as the vehicle that will carry you along that road. This introduction will cover some traditional concepts of marketing, and discuss how they can help you on your journey—and some of the hazards and detours along the highway that you need to watch out for.

Marketing can be defined as *any activity that you do that is meant to increase your business*. That may be everything from refining the message on your answering machine to handing out business cards to buying time on a television station. Advertising is simply marketing that you have to pay for. A successful therapist I know sums it up in one sentence: *Advertising is money going out; marketing is money coming in.*

If you read most marketing textbooks, you'll see that they all for the most part have a few things in common. They advise you to do a market study before starting a business. They advise you to identify your target market, and they tell you that in your first couple of years in business, you have to be prepared to spend 20–30% of your gross income on advertising, and they spend a lot of time talking about the attributes of the successful businessperson.

When I started my business, my market study consisted of looking in the phone book and driving around town to see how many other therapists were around and where they were located. My target market was *everybody.* Unless you want to have a real niche practice, such as only working on pregnant women, why would you want to exclude anyone from your target market? That concept doesn't work for me. As for advertising, 30% of my first year's budget wouldn't have paid for one impressive ad in a big city newspaper. I had to be creative, and spread my advertising dollars as thinly as possible. If you *do* have a niche practice, you can do marketing that is specific to a population if you choose to, but unless you *only* want to attract that population, you ought to act as if *everybody* in your area is a potential client.

Here are some examples: You take out an ad in a local magazine called *Suburban Woman.* You have just spent money to advertise exclusively to women, and that's okay—assuming you don't want any men for clients. Or you take out an ad in *North Carolina Hunting and Fishing*, and you'll get just the opposite effect—98% of the readers are male. Another illustration: You've discovered you can get some low-cost ads from your local television company—but if they only run during the breaks in the Sunday morning show from a local church, you have limited yourself to a relatively small audience—so the cost isn't as small as it seems. If you don't mind having clients that are young, old, male, female, rich, middle-class, or whatever, you want to market yourself to the general population of your area, and not just cater to a small faction of it. Choose advertising venues that will be seen by the general public.

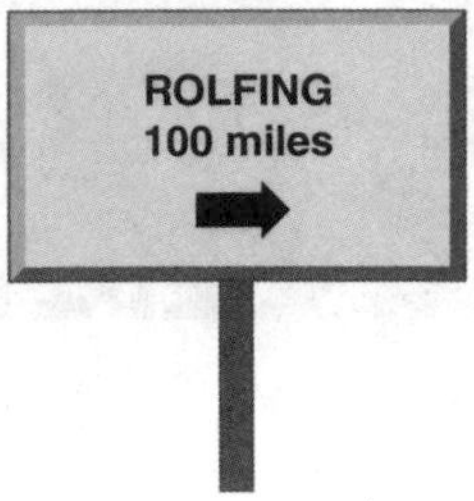

Another traditional principle of marketing is to advertise yourself most heavily within a certain radius of your business. While that may hold true for the therapist who is strictly doing Swedish massage or neuromuscular therapy, therapists who *do* have a specialty may want to capitalize on that and market themselves in surrounding areas as well. If you are the only person practicing Rolfing in a 100-mile radius, it may serve you to advertise in adjoining towns and cities. Don't limit yourself by defining your target market too narrowly.

By way of explanation, the four P's of marketing are product, price, place, and promotion. All you have to do is find the right combination—what will work for you in your unique situation—to get started on the path to increased prosperity.

The First P: Product

Massage therapy is a service business. As with any other service, the price, the place, and the promotion are all variables, but the product remains the same—whether you are trying to land your ideal job or establish your own business, the product is *you.*

You are either a professional massage therapist or on your way to becoming one. If you're still a student, look around at your classmates (discreetly, of course). What qualities would you say you have that would make a client, or an employer, choose you over someone else? If you're already practicing, ask yourself the same question. You are not just selling a massage, but a total experience that actually hinges on one thing—you. You are the product. Your personality, your communication skills, your level of service, your professional demeanor, the way you dress, even the cleanliness of your office, may be more important than your technical skills as a massage therapist when it comes to marketing yourself to a potential employer or to the public. Put yourself in the shoes of the client for a moment. What do *you* want when you visit a massage therapist? What do you want when paying for any service? *Service* is the key word.

Unless you're the only therapist in a small town, there's plenty of competition out there. You want someone who's sensitive to your needs, respectful of your time, treats you as if you're the most important client she has, gives you good value for the money, and is highly skilled. That's not much to ask, right?

Whether you are still in school or just need a breath of fresh air in your business, decide now that *you are a superior product* that must be marketed as such. On the other hand, don't lose sight of the fact that it doesn't matter what glorious attributes you possess if they're not marketed in the right way.

A Special Product: The Male Massage Therapist

It's not that a male therapist is any more special as a person than a female therapist, per se, but male therapists do have their own set of problems and considerations. Those considerations may vary depending on where you live and practice, and what type of work you do. As a male, you may have an easier time selling your services if you have a specialty—but don't despair if that's not the case.

If you're a male therapist just out of school, you may initially have an easier time getting established by working in a chiropractor's office, spa, or other group practice. Being a part of a group can also be a source of support to the therapist who is just starting out; the plan may be to strike out on your own in the future, but it might not hurt to gain some initial exposure by working in an office with others. If you're determined to jump right out of school into doing your own thing, there are a few caveats that apply to male therapists:

- Some females do not feel comfortable receiving bodywork from a male.
- There are lots of homophobic males who do not feel comfortable receiving bodywork from a male.
- Some females who would not mind receiving bodywork from a male have a spouse who does not want them to receive massage from a male.

If you are facing these facts at the outset, you can certainly overcome them through establishing yourself as a talented, knowledgeable, and professional-demeanored therapist that both male and female clients can feel comfortable with. The reasoning in suggesting starting out in a group practice is that a female might feel more comfortable receiving massage from a male therapist if there are other people around until she gets to know you.

Frankly, in my own situation I always feel caught between a rock and a hard place where male therapists are concerned. Among my dozen or so independent contractors, at any given time, there are one or two males. While I do not want to act as if it would be any different to receive a massage from a male than a female, I do not feel that I can surprise a teenage girl or an 80-year-old lady with the news that her massage therapist is a male after she has already arrived at the office expecting to receive her massage. When someone calls for an appointment, I will normally say something like, "Jennifer has an opening at 2 on Thursday, or Fred has an opening Friday at 10 am." That way, I am giving them a choice. It is okay to say "Are you comfortable with a male therapist?" I don't want to put a stigma on it; I just feel compelled to inform the client. In my own office, the male therapist who practices the Rolf Method® is much busier than the male who has a more general practice. In spite of the fact that the other young man is very good at massage, clean-cut and personable, he has never enjoyed the clientele that the female therapists have, and in fact supplements his income with other jobs as the need dictates. Males can and do make it in the massage business; it just takes perseverance and making their product stand out above the crowd; more about that in Chapter 5

The Second P: Price

We all want to make a good living doing something we enjoy. If you are working for a big company or even another individual, you may have no control over the price that's being charged for your services; you might be paid a flat hourly rate whether you are busy or not; you may be earning a commission on the work you do or the products you sell (yes, some places expect you to sell).

If, however, you are in business for yourself or intending to be, take time to carefully research and think through your pricing structure. It's wise to check out the other therapists in your area to see what they are charging, and be somewhat in line with that—depending on several factors. If you're in business for yourself and have many years of experience, you may feel perfectly justified (and rightly so) for charging more than someone who just graduated from massage school, but if you are working in someone else's business, it's likely that all therapists have the same pay scale regardless of experience.

If you have a plush office in a galleria adjacent to a ritzy neighborhood with million-dollar homes, you can charge more than the home office practitioner or the therapist who has a rented room in a less expensive part of town. Those practitioners may be lower on overhead; that doesn't mean their *time* is worth less that the person in the fancy office, but it does mean they're not forced to charge a premium price for premium surroundings.

If the other therapists in your area are charging between $50–$60 per hour, and you are only charging $25, or you are charging $90, there ought to be a good explanation for that. If you're on the lower end of that, you are either a) serving the poor, b) you have a low sense of self-worth, or c) you're trying to take business away from other therapists by undercutting their prices. If you're serving the poor—maybe you feel called to massage only senior citizens on limited incomes—go right ahead and ignore any nay-saying, and kudos to you. If you don't think you're worth as much as everyone else, why not? Aren't you well-trained? Don't you have confidence in your ability to help people relax or get them out of pain? You have to cultivate self-confidence if you're lacking in that area, and working for slave wages isn't going to instill it in you. Charge what you're worth! And if you're working cheaply just to undercut other therapists to try to take business away from them, shame on you. That's a shabby tactic better left to unscrupulous salesmen. Charging a fair price and giving a good value for the money is acting with integrity—and always a good business practice.

On the other side, if your office surroundings are comparable to other therapists in the area, charging a lot more than other therapists, especially when you're first starting out, is probably not a good idea unless you have a really good reason why—and one that you can publicize as the reason you're worth more, such as "each session is an hour and a half; I feel I need that much time to accomplish the work I want to do with people," or some other plausible excuse.

If you're self-employed, your pricing structure is also an important part of your total budget, and will be key in determining how much money you can spend on marketing. Bear in mind, the cost of anything can vary greatly from place to place—the cost of a massage, and the costs associated with doing business. I live in a small town in North Carolina. An hour to the west, the price of everything is much higher than it is here, because it's a mountain tourist area where you pay a premium for the view. If you live in a small rural town in South Dakota, you are going to be able to operate (and market yourself) more cheaply than the therapist who lives in Manhattan. At the same time, the therapist who lives and works in Manhattan will probably be charging substantially more for a massage than the one in South Dakota.

Your Unique Situation

Your pricing structure and your advertising budget will depend on your unique situation. If you have decided to work out of your home, strictly on a referral basis, you may not even want your number published in the phone book, nor desire to have any advertising at all. You may feel you'll get all the customers you want through word-of-mouth.

If you are working in someone else's clinic setting, you may not have any input into the advertising. I once worked in a clinic with seven or eight other therapists, and the owner never did any advertising for the clinic. The therapists banded together and wanted to buy some nice ads, at our shared expense, with a group picture and a listing of our specialties, and the owner vetoed it. He wanted it to be all about his clinic instead of any of us as individuals—the very people who made the place what it was. There are some good questions to ask the owner of any business you are thinking of working in—do you advertise, where do you advertise, will I be expected to or prohibited from advertising myself, is any self-advertising encouraged or prohibited, and so forth—before you accept a job. If they aren't willing to answer those questions, go elsewhere to work.

The Third P: Place

Location, Location, Location

We've mentioned a few possibilities in the previous sections about place, and how that will affect your budget, your pricing, and your marketing plans. Let's talk about actual physical place in its own context for a moment.

An upstairs office is *never* a good idea, unless there is an elevator. An upstairs office with no elevator immediately removes physically handicapped people from your list of potential clients, and others won't like it either, including people with limited mobility due to age, injury, or other pathology; people with sciatica or other leg or hip problems may not enjoy climbing a long flight of stairs, and so forth.

Therapists who work in a home office need to be particularly mindful of presenting a professional image. Be sure clients don't have to trip over toys on the floor on their way to the massage table or the bathroom. Think it over carefully, and weigh all sides. Some therapists want to work at home for just that reason—to be a stay-at-home mom, and that's admirable, but if your children are at home and still of screaming age, a home office may not be your best shot for success. It may be better for you to schedule clients during the afternoon nap period or in the evenings after the little ones have gone to bed. Another consideration: most homes are not set up for handicapped access—another limitation to your practice. There may also be zoning restrictions against operating a business in your home, depending on where you live. Be sure you operate within the laws of your locality.

When choosing office space, be realistic about what you can afford, while at the same time being mindful that location is important. My own office, while still on Main Street, is just south of the main part of town, not right in the most congested part of town. I could have gotten an office for half the price that I pay now just a few blocks up the street, but we have a horrible parking problem in that area of our town, and the places on the sidewalk for handicapped access are few and far between. Keep those things in mind when you're looking for a place.

Be mindful of the area you choose. If your town has such establishments, you do not want an office next door to a bar, strip club, adult bookstore, or anyplace else that has sexual connotations, loud music, or other loud noise. You wouldn't want to be located next door to a metal fabrication shop where the main noise is a hammer banging on steel, for instance.

On the other hand, an office in or near a medical complex is a great place if you practice medical massage. Some municipalities, unfortunately, have not caught on to the fact that massage is not about sex and still have barbaric zoning restrictions on "massage parlors." Again, investigate any zoning laws or business restrictions before signing a lease.

Choose your location carefully. While there's certainly nothing wrong with "moving up" into a bigger and/or nicer space, you should ideally establish yourself in a place you intend to remain for a long time. And unless you are only working for someone else for a time in order to save money toward the goal of opening your own place, it's also wise to settle into a job that you hopefully will remain at for a long time as well, if that's the road you're taking. Again, there's nothing wrong with moving up to a better job if it means a nicer place, more money, or better benefits; but if you have the intent of building up a steady clientele, it's hard to do that if you're changing jobs every few months. While some clients might be glad to follow you from place to place, others will remain at a business that's closer to their home, or that perhaps they have loyalty to the owner of the establishment rather than to you. I happen to like a particular hairdresser in our town, and I have followed her to several different salons. However, when she decided to move for the fourth time, I finally decided to just stick with the last salon she was at, which was conveniently right up the street from my office.

"Job-hopping" also does not look good to future employers, in case you're out there looking. Many employers would jump to the conclusion that someone who has been at several places in the space of a year or two is not worth hiring. If they get the impression you're just going to stay long enough to find the next best thing, they may not be willing to invest time and money in training you to do things their way. They might also assume that you have a problem getting along with people. If you have had a number of jobs in a relatively short period of time, be prepared at a job interview to answer questions about why you have moved around so much.

The Fourth P: Promotion

The remainder of this book is devoted to promotion. Are you aware that fear of success is the very same thing as fear of failure? It's all a fear of *change*. Jumping into something new is exciting and scary at the same time, but it's usually the unknown that scares us. Defining your goals sets the stage for *positive* change, and is the first week's activity in Chapter 2. By setting your goals, you are taking the first step to mapping out your course to prosperity. Be diligent with your journaling. It will help you keep focused on your financial and personal goals. Promotion is going to be second nature to you a year from now.

The Ethics of Promotion

This isn't meant to be an ethics book; it's a marketing book, so I am only going to talk about ethics as they relate to marketing your business, with one added caveat: if you don't conduct yourself ethically, all the marketing tricks in the world aren't going to help you. Acting unethically will catch up with you, and usually sooner than later. That said, let's take a look at a Code of Ethics and see how that affects the promotion of your massage and bodywork services. The American Massage Therapy Association (AMTA), the National Certification Board for Therapeutic Massage & Bodywork (NCBTMB), and other national organizations and state boards have their own codes, and they are similar in many ways. The following Code of Ethics is the Code from NCBTMB:

Massage and Bodywork Therapists shall act in a manner that justifies public trust and confidence, enhances the reputation of the profession, and safeguards the interest of individual clients. To this end, massage and bodywork therapists in the exercise of accountability will:

I. Have a sincere commitment to provide the highest quality of care to those who seek their professional services.

II. Represent their qualifications honestly, including education and professional affiliations, and provide only those services that they are qualified to perform.

III. Accurately inform clients, other health care practitioners, and the public of the scope and limitations of their discipline.
IV. Acknowledge the limitations of and contraindications for massage and bodywork and refer clients to appropriate health professionals.
V. Provide treatment only where there is reasonable expectation that it will be advantageous to the client.
VI. Consistently maintain and improve professional knowledge and competence, striving for professional excellence through regular assessment of personal and professional strengths and weaknesses and through continued education training.
VII. Conduct their business and professional activities with honesty and integrity, and respect the inherent worth of all persons.
VIII. Refuse to unjustly discriminate against clients or health professionals.
IX. Safeguard the confidentiality of all client information, unless disclosure is required by law or necessary for the protection of the public.
X. Respect the client's right to treatment with informed and voluntary consent. The certified practitioner will obtain and record the informed consent of the client, or client's advocate, before providing treatment. This consent may be written or verbal.
XI. Respect the client's right to refuse, modify, or terminate treatment regardless of prior consent given.
XII. Provide draping and treatment in a way that ensures the safety, comfort and privacy of the client.
XIII. Exercise the right to refuse to treat any person or part of the body for just and reasonable cause.
XIV. Refrain, under all circumstances, from initiating or engaging in any sexual conduct, sexual activities, or sexualizing behavior involving a client, even if the client attempts to sexualize the relationship.
XV. Avoid any interest, activity or influence which might be in conflict with the practitioner's obligation to act in the best interests of the client or the profession.
XVI. Respect the client's boundaries with regard to privacy, disclosure, exposure, emotional expression, beliefs, and the client's reasonable expectations of professional behavior. Practitioners will respect the client's autonomy.
XVII. Refuse any gifts or benefits that are intended to influence a referral, decision or treatment, or that are purely for personal gain and not for the good of the client.
XVIII. Follow all policies, procedures, guidelines, regulations, codes, and requirements promulgated by the National Certification Board for Therapeutic Massage and Bodywork.

Let's examine the Code as a guideline for marketing.

- Article I: Of course we have a desire and a commitment to provide our clients with the highest level of service we are capable of, and we should feel free to advertise that fact.
- Articles II, III, IV, and V: We could say that all these pertain to truth in advertising. Represent yourself and your qualifications honestly, don't advertise that you do work you aren't qualified to do—and don't attempt to do work you aren't qualified to do. Refer people when necessary. As you'll find out in Chapter 18, those referral opportunities are beneficial to everyone concerned.

- Article VI: Every time you fulfill your desire and/or obligation to get continuing education, you are gaining new skills that you can promote.
- Article VII: Conduct your business with honesty and integrity; if you do otherwise, no amount of advertising will help you—particularly in a small town, the word will get around.
- Article VIII: Marketing to everyone and viewing everyone as a potential client and/or potential source of referrals is the way to maximize success. Discriminating is not.
- Article XI: Just like Article VII, if you blab about your clients, the word will get around. Client testimonials are a great form of no-cost marketing—and you must have their permission.
- Articles X–XVIII: all pertain to conducting ourselves with ethical behavior and respecting client boundaries.

States that license massage therapists and have their own code of ethics may place specific limitations or rules on the advertisement and marketing of massage therapy. In our state, for instance, our code states that any advertising, including signage, business cards, print ads, radio ads, and so forth must include the license number of the therapist. Be sure that you abide by any and all codes and laws that you are subject to.

PART 1

Mapping Out Your Journey

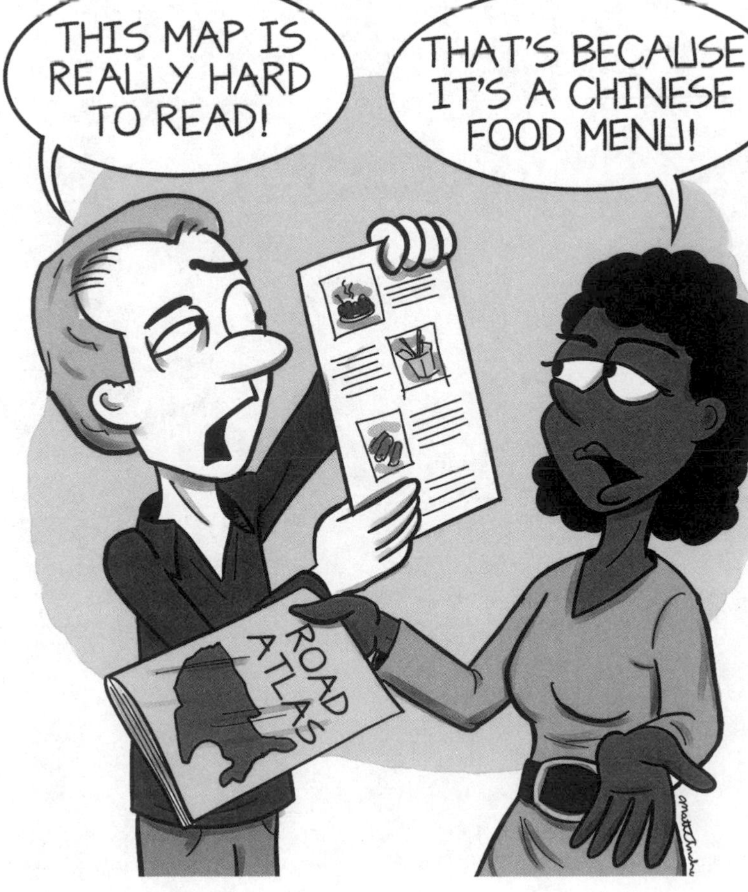

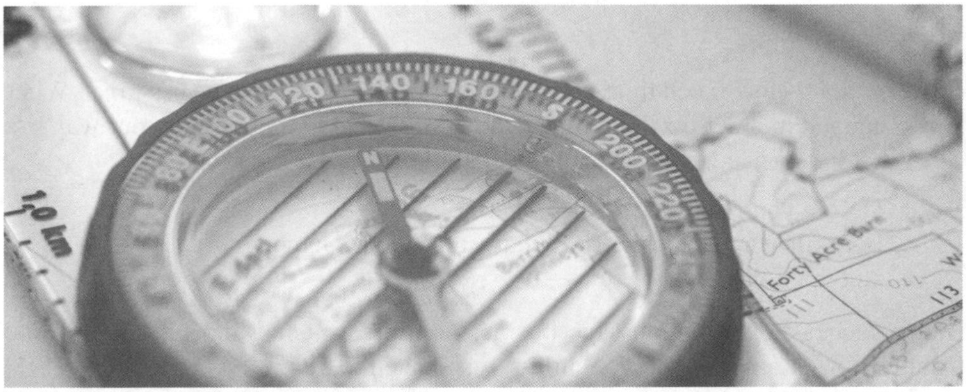

CHAPTER 1

Defining Your Goals

You've achieved success in your field when you don't know whether what you're doing is work or play.

—Warren Beatty

Your goals are as individual as you are. Ask almost any businessperson what her goals are, and it usually comes down to one thing, regardless of how it's worded: *to succeed.* Your definition of success may be to have so many clients you have to turn them away, while your fellow therapist may think it's enough money to get by and plenty of spare time to go fishing.

Your goals are an important part of not only your marketing plan, but your overall business plan. If your goal is to work from your home office so that you can stay home with your young children, your plan is going to be quite a bit different from the therapist who wants to work towards owning a ritzy spa in an exotic tourist destination, or the therapist who desires a steady nine-to-five position in a chiropractor's office.

Patti's Story

My Story

When I entered massage school, I already knew that I wanted to work at home. I didn't wait for graduation to start planning and cultivating my practice. I set up my massage table in my spare room and turned it into my massage space. I had fun decorating and making it into a nice, serene space. Whenever I felt comfortable enough with the clients I met during school clinic days, I would give them a coupon for a free massage that had a map to my house printed on the back along with my home phone number. Five years later, many of these same people are still my clients.

Writing down your goals gives you a more concrete sense of them than idly daydreaming about things you want to happen "someday." Where would you like to be a year from now, or five years from now? How much money do you want to earn per year? How much time off from work do you want in a year's time? What has to happen in order for these things to occur? What is standing in your way?

What has to happen in order for these things to occur is for you to:

- Define your goals.
- Formulate a plan designed to make those goals happen.
- Act upon that plan.

Being successful in the massage business requires mental and physical effort. Clients won't drop into your lap unless you shake the tree.

If you have defined your goals and have some good ideas, but haven't put them into place yet, resolve to stop procrastinating right now. As stated in the Introduction, fear of success is the very same thing as fear of failure—it's all *fear of change*. Thinking big and planning for success beyond your wildest dreams can seem like a scary thing—especially when you realize it's all up to you to make it happen. If you haven't yet written your business plan, or written down your professional goals if you're planning to work as someone else's employee, don't put it off any longer.

If you're just about to graduate from massage school, and want to be self-employed, your one-year plan might look similar to this example.

One-Year Plan

1. Take necessary exams and obtain licenses.
2. Open a business savings account.
3. Spend one year working in nearby resort spa in order to save money to rent own office space.
4. Scout for good locations; notice how many other therapists are in area.
5. Gather information from the Small Business Administration (SBA), Chamber of Commerce, utility companies, supply companies, and advertising sources as background information in order to begin writing business plan and budgeting.

My goal for last year was to gain 365 new clients—one for each day. Since we're closed on Sunday, that meant that on another day during the week, we had to get two. This was not a secret plan. I shared it with all the other therapists on staff. I wrote the magic number on a sticky note and put it on my computer monitor where I would be sure to see it every day. With every new client, I would say to myself, "Thank you. 100 down; only 265 more to go." I thought about it every day. I gave it a voice every day by telling the other staff members how we were doing. At the end of the year, we had actually gained 480, an amazing feat in an economically depressed small town of about 20,000 residents that not only had a number of other therapists but a massage school with a student clinic as well.

A prerequisite for goal-setting is to have a positive attitude. I *believed* we could get those clients. My staff believed it. I believed if I acted successful, I would be successful. Thought is the most powerful thing in the universe. If you expect to fail, you've taken your first step on the way to failure. You have to believe in yourself and your abilities. We all know that massage is a great product. To borrow a phrase from Estée Lauder: "If your product isn't selling, the problem isn't the product, it's *you*."

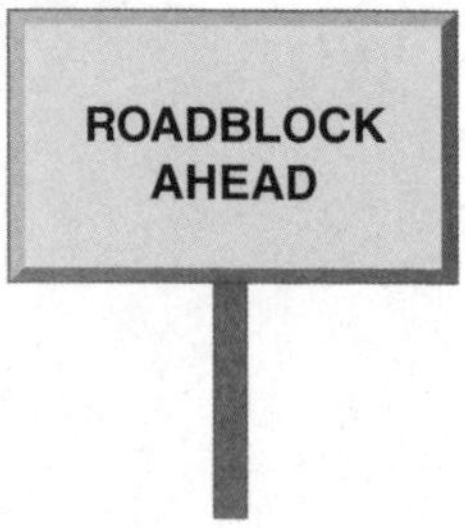

Not only is a positive attitude important to goal-setting, it is important to your clients. No one wants to visit a person who's negative and whiny. People want to see a therapist who will make them feel good and who will act happy while doing it.

Some healthy introspection is called for—especially if you're an old hand who has been doing massage for a while and still haven't met your income and other career goals. Whatever we allow to get in our way, will get in our way. We all have obligations we have to meet; we all have choices to make. If you have to pick up your child at school at 3:00 and have him at soccer practice at 4:00, that's an obligation. If you are sitting in your office playing solitaire on the computer instead of working on marketing your business, that's a choice—and a poor one, unless you have all the business you desire.

Remember the old adage, "the early bird gets the worm"? That's true. Most people have to work for what they get, and unless your family owns Standard Oil or J.C. Penney, so do you. It's easy to fall into a stagnant place. You have to work at it to keep that from happening. That's not to say you shouldn't have downtime—to play solitaire or whatever your particular stress relief is—but don't fall into a trap. The single biggest mistake new massage therapists make is sitting in the office waiting for business to come to them. While you're writing down your goals, it will be helpful to you to write down what is getting in the way of your ideal practice, as well. Maybe you're waiting until you have enough money for expensive advertising. You don't have to. The rest of this book will be filled with no-cost and low-cost ways to promote yourself.

My Personal Journey

This Week's Activity: Defining My Goals Date ____________

This week, take the time to define what it is you want: what type of work situation you hope to be in when you get your license, what kind of income you hope to make, what benefits you hope to have, how much time you want to spend at work and how much time you want to play. Define what it is that will make *you* feel successful as a massage therapist.

My Goals

____

____

____

What's in my way?

____

____

____

What action can I take to remedy the situation?

____

____

____

One-Year Progress Update Date ____________

____

____

____

POSITIVE AFFIRMATION: **I am on my way to success.**

CHAPTER 2

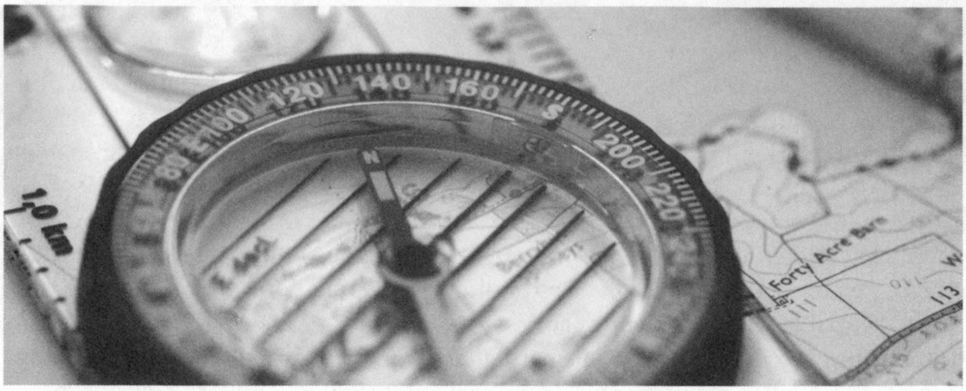

Your Marketing Budget

A successful individual typically sets his next goal somewhat but not too much above his last achievement. In this way he steadily raises his level of aspiration.

— Kurt Lewin

Now that you have set your goals, it's time to create a marketing budget. Your marketing budget is going to be based on several factors. When constructing an overall budget for your business, the first things to account for are the things that you must have in order to operate your business: rent, electricity, water, and so forth. Once you see how much money it takes just to operate, you'll have a better idea of how much money you can spend on marketing. And remember, advertising is going to be just one piece—and hopefully, a small one—of your marketing pie. The more free and low-cost marketing opportunities you take advantage of, the more will be left over for you to save or spend on other things.

If this is your first year in business, you don't have any past history to help you make budget projections. You may have to do a little research. If you call the power company, they will tell you what the average power bill has been for your office in the past couple of years, so you can make a good estimate. Same with the water company, and of course if you have agreed to pay $500 a month in rent, you can quickly figure out that comes to $6,000 per year. Remember, as we stated in the Introduction, there will be quite a variance in the cost of goods and services, depending on where you live. Commercial spaces tend to be rented (or sold) based on square footage. Here in my town, you can rent 1,000 square feet—the minimum space you could have a comfortable massage room in, not counting any lobby or reception area—as cheaply as $200 per month. In New York, $200 wouldn't pay for a small closet. Investigate as many options as you can before deciding where to hang your shingle.

A little more difficult is projecting how much revenue you are going to have. The all-important figure you need to know is your break-even point. How many massages do you have to do just to pay the bills? The monthly budget for my own business looks like this.

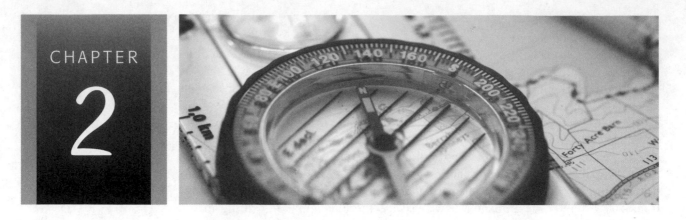

Sample Monthly Budget

Rent $1,450
Telephone/Internet service $370
Electricity/gas $230
Water $90
Bottled water service $50
Insurance $30 (I pay it annually, but this is the monthly breakdown)
Laundry expenses $100 (detergent, dryer sheets, bleach)
Office supplies $150
Janitorial supplies $50
Yellow Pages ad $90
Cleaning service $80
Monthly total $2,690

I have over a dozen independent contractors working out of my office, so my situation may be very different from yours, but the formula is the same: add up all of your costs, and then figure how many massages you have to do, at what price, to find your break-even point. The prices of the services here vary, but at an average price of $50 per service, we have to do 54 massages just to break even. Notice that this budget did not include *anything* set aside for advertising, with the exception of my Yellow Pages ad. I also have a couple of expenses listed that everyone may not need. The water in our town tastes like chlorine to me, so I purchase bottled water for our clients. I also do the daily cleaning here myself; the $80 per month set aside for cleaning is the average cost of having my carpets cleaned once every three months—something I barter for (but am still paying the therapists to perform; more about that in Chapter 29). I don't have anything budgeted for maintenance and repairs because (handily) my husband is a builder, and I depend on him to fix anything that goes wrong. Everyone is not so lucky!

Ricky's Story

My Story

Massage is my second career. I intend to move to a bigger city 40 miles away when I retire from my day job in two years. For the past year, I have advertised outcalls in the monthly city magazine and I have a small listing in the Yellow Pages. I got a great rate for committing to a year's worth of ads in the magazine, and that's the only advertising I am doing for now. I usually make the drive three or four nights a week and do at least two massages each night as a result of the ads, and the referrals my customers are sending me. My schedule is a little exhausting for now, but I feel I am building my business and will be established by the time I am ready to make the move. I'm willing to do whatever it takes to make a go of it.

How much should you budget for marketing? As stated in the Introduction, traditional marketing theories advise that a new, start-up business should plan to spend 20% to 30% of gross income marketing during the first couple of years. The best thing to do is cut that as low as possible by using no-cost and low-cost marketing strategies that will get your name out to the public without the big expense. When constructing your budget, look for ways to cut costs in other areas (without hurting service to the client, of course) so that you can spend advertising dollars where they are most important—a Yellow Pages ad, for instance. Each year, I go through my budget with a fine-toothed comb and look for expenses that are out of control, and find a course of action to remedy the situation. I'll use my laundry situation as a good example.

For the past couple of years, I have been using a national laundry service that has competitive pricing. Even though they were reasonable, I have been spending more than $500 per month for linen service. And they were only providing sheets; that doesn't count the towels and pillowcases that I was taking home nightly to wash.

I'm also an educator, and along with the laundry expense, I had also been paying $140 per day for a conference room at a local hotel where I could hold my twice-monthly classes (which, incidentally, I had to clean myself, or pay extra money for cleaning). Add that together with the laundry expense, and that's $780 per month. Recently, the office next door to mine became vacant. It rents for $725 per month. I rented that space, the landlord agreed to reconfigure the office for me to include a laundry room, and the rest of it is my wide-open classroom space that accommodates just as many students as I had at the hotel. I invested in 50 pairs of sheets and a nice washer and dryer, and am now coming out ahead every month. I have to spend an hour or so a day on laundry, and replace the sheets occasionally, but even so, I'm better off financially and time-wise. I no longer have to haul things to the hotel to teach classes or take the towels home at night. And I'm able to rent the room out to other teachers and offer classes to the community as well. In addition to the continuing education we offer for massage therapists, we're now offering yoga, t'ai chi, belly dancing, raw food classes, and other education to the general public. The room is paying for itself.

Other hidden costs are related to personal spending habits. That $4 cappuccino on the way to work every morning adds up to $80 a month—which would pay for an ad every month (or at least be a partial payment, if you live in a big city with expensive ad rates). Eating lunch out every day equals a half-page ad in my local newspaper. Financial experts often recommend that in order to figure out where you're really spending your money, carry around a little notebook for a month and write down every single penny you spend, whether it's cash, check, or credit card—and they can almost always guarantee that at the end of that month, you'll be shocked to see where a lot of your money is really going. A little here, a little there, adds up to much more than you might realize.

Office and janitorial supplies are purchased at the cheapest price possible. I use end-tab file folders for my client files, and the manila ones are about $35 per box. Recently while I was in the office supply store, the sale rack had five boxes that were on sale for $7 a box because they were various colors that hadn't been selling. I bought five boxes for what I normally pay for one—it doesn't matter to me, or the client, if they're funky colors, they work just the same. Thrift stores and yard sales are often good sources for miscellaneous office items. I purchase janitorial supplies such as cleaners and paper towels at one of those stores where everything in the store is $1. They're not name brands, but they work just the same as the items that are three times the price if purchased at the grocery store. By cutting your budget in as many areas as possible, that leaves more left for the advertising that *is* necessary, not to mention more to go into your pocket.

Wasting Your Advertising Dollars

Because not all marketing can be accomplished at no or low cost, you want to have a certain amount of money budgeted for the advertising that you really want to do—things like nice signage, the Yellow Pages, and so forth. In order to have that money, there are some types of advertising that you are going to have to avoid. Here are some advertising opportunities that you should run—not walk—away from. If your son hits you up to buy a $50 ad on his Little League calendar, or your mother wants you to buy an ad in her church cookbook, you are of course going to do it if you have the money, even if it means not advertising somewhere else where that money would be better spent. We are not talking about those instances.

We are talking about the constant barrage of advertising "opportunities" that come our way. The Little League calendar and church cookbooks are only a couple of examples, along with having your ad in school annuals, telephone book covers, football programs, and the like. If you don't have a personal investment like your child or your mother breathing down your neck to buy an ad, pass on these. Always stack up *how much you are spending against possible return from the ad.*

I recently got a call from a company that wanted to sell me a business card-sized ad on the telephone book cover. She quoted me the price of $350 and said that they would only feature one business of each kind on the cover, so mine would be the only local massage business with an ad on the cover. The figures started ticking in my head—I'm thinking 40,000 plus residents in our county, reach them all for $350, when it occurred to me to ask her exactly how many copies would be distributed, at which point she confessed that she was talking about 1,000 covers for $350. It wasn't such a good deal, after all. For the same $350, I can get a half-page ad in the newspaper that will in fact reach 40,000 people. It's a much better value for the money. But wait—a client who is a real estate agent told me the same company approached him to buy an ad—and gave him the ad for no charge because he agreed to distribute the phone book. That didn't take much effort on his part, just giving them away in his office and carrying a few at a time in the car to give away whenever he was showing property. Now that I know that, next time that company calls me, I'll ask them if I can distribute for them in exchange for a free ad. I don't have anything to lose by asking, and the answer might be *yes*.

Another therapist I know paid $500 to have her ad on the prescription drug bags given out at a local drugstore. They guaranteed her it would be on at least 10,000 bags in a year's time. This particular company solicited discount coupons to go on the bags, so she put a "$10 off on massage" coupon on the bag. She failed to specify that she wanted to limit that to new customers only. This therapist practiced near a retirement community, and had cultivated a business of primarily seniors, many of whom are on prescription drugs. She redeemed a lot of the coupons, after a rather rude awakening. A weekly client came in with a coupon and presented it at the end of the massage. The therapist said to her that they were only for first-time clients, and the client became indignant and told her that she should have specified that on the coupon—which was true, and the therapist was forced to relent. The bottom line of it was the woman was taking multiple prescriptions and she saved up enough coupons—no expiration date or "one to a customer" on them either—to receive her massages $10 cheaper for many months to come. She alone counted for a $40 monthly reduction in the therapist's pay, and she wasn't the only regular customer redeeming the coupons. Put careful thought into participating in such promotions, and make sure you can afford the participation.

I might add here that I advertise on prescription drug bags from a certain drugstore myself. This is not an advertising venue I would normally choose to participate in, and it was my third year in business before I began to do so. There are several reasons I am spending my advertising dollars there. This is not a chain store, it is a locally owned business on Main Street; the three partners who are the owners all patronize my business regularly, and for every occasion that they have a need to give someone a gift, they buy them a gift certificate from my business. They have more than 60 employees, and at least 10 of them are clients, referred by the owners. In a year's time, they are contributing a minimum of $6,000 to my coffers. The ad that I place on their prescription bags cost $260 per year and they guarantee that my ad will be on a minimum of 24,000 bags. I don't have any discount offers on the ad; it's just an ad with the bare facts of what we do and our contact information. Because it costs me the equivalent of less than five massages per year to pay for, it's a good deal for me—based on the circumstances.

School annuals are usually passed around at school for a week or so with kids signing each other's books, and then they are put on the shelf where they remain in obscurity until the kids are grown and move into their own place, at which point they're packed in a box and may never be seen again—another waste of advertising dollars. Again, if your child isn't putting a guilt trip on you, don't buy those ads.

Advertising as a sponsor of a local sports team, dance team, or something similar is also usually a poor return for advertising dollars. Say you buy a sign for $500 that will stay on the football field for one year. The football team plays 20 games a season. But wait . . . half of those games are played away. Of the ten that are played there, one of those teams is from elsewhere—not your community. Depending on how big your local high school is, the ad might be seen by anywhere from 50 to 5,000 people. At least half of those are the high school students themselves, most of whom are not yet massage clients. You may get *some* business from the parents who are present and see your ad. Again, stack up possible return against the cost of the ad. Your ad may be seen by 5,000 people, but if 4,000 of them are minors, realistically that is 1,000 potential customers you will reach instead of 5,000. That breaks down to a cost of $0.50 per person, not a very good advertising rate.

Advertising that reaches a very limited audience is rarely a good producer of revenue. It may be nice of you to buy a $100 ad to place on the program of the play that the arts council is producing. But if past experience shows that those plays are usually attended by 100 people or less, it isn't a good deal. Also, a play program is going to be looked at the night of the play, and quite possibly thrown in the trash on the way out the door after the performance. Unless a person collects those, it's one of those pieces of paper that tends to wind up in a pile or a drawer with other "important" papers until it's finally thrown away.

Ads on placemats and menus in restaurants are another opportunity that must be looked at carefully. Usually, the restaurant itself does not have anything to do with these ads. The ad company convinces a restaurant that they can get their menus and placemats for free by selling advertising on them, and of course the ad company is the one that makes a big fat fee. Before you purchase one of these, gather some information. Is the restaurant close to your business, or 15 miles away? Is it a popular place, or is it struggling and may be closed by the time your menus are printed? How many customers do they serve in a week, a month, a year? Will the ad be on takeout menus as well? Who makes up their customer base? Is it a situation such as my drugstore bags, where the owners and employees are loyal customers of yours?

Once you have gathered that information, add it up to see if you think it will give you a good return. If it's a diner that caters to minimum-wage factory employees in a depressed area where unemployment is running high—you will probably not see much return on the investment. If it's a popular lunch spot in the middle of the business district, patronized by lawyers, other professionals, and office workers—maybe so. The second group is apt to have more discretionary income to spend on things like massage. One caveat: If you should decide to advertise on restaurant menus, it is very wise to contact the restaurant owner before placing the ad, in spite of the fact that the restaurant is usually not involved in the actual selling of the ad space. Just check in with them, to make sure that they have in fact approved of the menus and the timeline, and that they know the company selling the ads to be reputable. I had a bad experience with something like this just a few months ago. Someone called me to solicit an ad, and the restaurant they were soliciting for was owned by people who are clients of my business and who have sent a number of customers to me. Based on those facts, I decided to place the ad. As it turns out, so much time had passed between the ad company approaching this restaurant about their menus, and the actual delivery of the menus, that the restaurant owners had implemented a number of price increases and changes in their menu, and they tossed those new menus right in the trash can when they finally arrived—no loss to them since they hadn't paid for them; the advertisers had. I lost the $125 I had paid for an ad. There was no recourse because there had been no date of guaranteed delivery, and I didn't want to complain to the owners as they are such good customers. It was one of life's little lessons.

To summarize, if you have the money to spare, you should advertise anywhere and everywhere that it makes you feel good—even if that means supporting every kid activity, school event, church cookbook, and the like that comes your way. But if you are in the position of needing to budget your advertising dollars, the objective is to get as much bang for the buck as possible. You can figure it out by using this formula.

Advertising Formula

4 × 6 Ad in the Newspaper

Cost of ad: $300. Divide by circulation: 50,000.
Cost per person of the ad: $0.006.

4 × 6 Ad on the Football Calendar

Cost of ad: $200. Divide by circulation: 5,000.
Cost per person of the ad: $0.04.

Obviously, the ad in the paper reaches many more people, at a much lower cost per person, and thus gives you more for your advertising dollar.

A budget isn't always easy to stick to. It requires discipline. Avoid the temptation to use credit cards for your advertising. You don't want to be paying off the ad in last Sunday's paper a year from now. Filling in the blanks on the sample budget (Table 2.1) will assist you in figuring out a marketing budget. You will notice that advertising is the last expense listed. That's because if you don't take care of the other bills first, you won't need to worry about advertising your business. The last column is for you to compare your actual figures at year's end so you will know whether you were reasonably accurate with your estimations.

Now let's figure out your projected income (Table 2.2). Ideally, you intend to do 25 massages per week (100 per month) at $60 each. That is $6,000 per month. How much does that leave you after you have paid your expenses? What does that do to your plan? If you follow the traditional marketing plan of spending 30% of your first-year gross income on advertising, that would mean $2,000 per month—a very hefty sum. However, remember that getting 25 clients a week is your best-case scenario. What if you're sick and don't work for two weeks? What if you only get 10 clients one week instead of 25; will you still be able to

Table 2.1 Sample Budget

Expense	Projected Monthly Cost	Total for Year	Actual Cost (Year End)
Rent			
Telephone/ Internet service			
Electricity/gas			
Water			
Insurance			
Laundry			
Office supplies			
Janitorial supplies			
Repairs/maintenance			
Miscellaneous			
Advertising			
TOTALS			

pay your bills? What if you truly work at marketing by using the low-cost and no-cost methods in this book and that $2,000 per month gets to go in your pocket instead?

Using this table along with your budget each month will help you recognize expenses that may be out of control. Have you ever noticed how many businesses, of any kind, open up and then are out of business within a few short months? That is because of unrealistic expectations people have that they're going to be drawing a salary and making a good living a couple of months down the road. My advice is to be prepared to work for a year before you start realizing any real income from your business. The premise of this book is that by following these principles for a year, you can start having a thriving practice; but do bear in mind that you are going to have start-up expenses during that year that are just that, one-time expenses such as utility and rent deposits, equipment and office purchases, and so forth. Be prepared to bite the bullet financially while you get your business up and running. Don't get a defeatist attitude—just a realistic one. At the end of my first year, when I looked at the one-time expenses of getting my practice off the ground, furnishing

Table 2.2 Projected Income

Projected Monthly Income (Gross)	**Actual Monthly Income**
Minus Projected Monthly Expenses	**Minus Actual Monthly Expenses**
Net Income	

my office, paying deposits, and the like, I found $14,000 that I would not have to spend the second year. If you're not good at organizing your finances, ask for help, and sooner rather than later. This is something you have to be brutally honest with yourself about. Somewhere in your town is a good CPA who'll be willing to trade her services for massage!

My Personal Journey

This Week's Activity: Working Out My Budget Date ____________________

For this week's activity, try working out the budget for your first year in business. If you intend to work as someone else's employee, do this anyway as a practice exercise. Use the forms on pages 11 and 12, create your own, or you may have similar forms from a business textbook you'd like to use. Make your income projections as well, based on your goals and ideals.

My Goals

___

___

___

What's in my way?

___

___

___

What action can I take to remedy the situation?

___

___

___

One-Year Progress Update Date ____________________

___

___

___

POSITIVE AFFIRMATION: **I live abundantly within my budget.**

CHAPTER

3

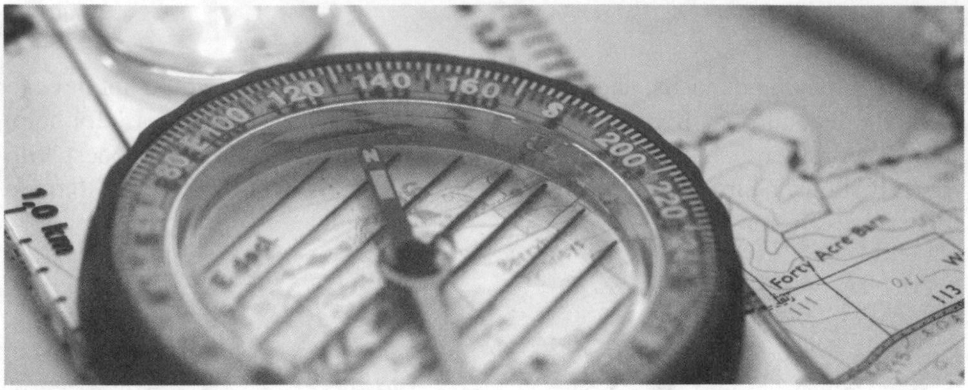

Developing Your Marketing Calendar

Success is not the result of spontaneous combustion. You must set yourself on fire.

—Reggie Leach

In conjunction with your marketing budget, it's a wise idea to plan on a marketing calendar. Once you have budgeted a certain amount of money for advertising, use the calendar as a tool to help you decide where you are going to spend it. In the course of a year, obvious opportunities for marketing massage packages and gift certificates are Christmas, Valentine's Day, Mother's Day, and Father's Day. Don't overlook Grandparent's Day and Secretary's Day. There are dozens of others that aren't as obvious. If you live in a town that is ethnically diverse, you may want to market some of the other culturally unique holidays: Kwanza, Hanukah, Chinese New Year, or St. Patrick's Day, for instance. There are also dozens of days that commemorate a historical event but are not officially holidays, and plenty of religious observance days.

Many observances last a week or a month; for instance February is Black History Month. March is American Red Cross Month. Consider hosting a blood drive at your office and giving a short chair massage to everyone who donates blood. April is Stress Awareness Month. May is Fibromyalgia Education and Awareness Month. Consider doing a free seminar on fibromyalgia. Invite some of your clients with fibromyalgia to come and speak about how they cope with their symptoms—because one of those ways is massage, and they're going to tell people that. September is Healthy Aging Month, a good month to target senior citizens with your promotions. October is Self-Promotion Month, *so promote yourself.*

MAY						
		1	2	3	4	5
6	7	8	9	10	11	12
13	14	15	16	17	18	19
20	21	22	23	24	25	26
27	28	29	30	31		

Your clients all have a birthday. I collect that information on my intake form. At the beginning of each month, I send a postcard to everyone who has a birthday during that month with an offer of a free paraffin hand treatment with their massage. I get dozens of these back every year. It's not only demonstrating customer appreciation for the regulars, but it sometimes serves to draw someone back in who hasn't been here in a while. For the first few years I was in business, I sent $5 off coupons for birthdays. The paraffin costs me a lot less money and is still a popular draw.

Be creative! Besides your clients' birthdays, you could have a promotion built around the birthday of a famous person. Alexander Hamilton's birthday is January 11 (in case you don't remember sixth grade history, Alexander Hamilton was the first secretary of the treasury, and his likeness is on ten dollar bills). Try offering a day of $10 chair massage on his birthday or something similar.

Each day, week, and month of the year, there is a holiday going on. I obtained this information from several websites that list obscure and silly holidays, and some that are not so silly. The month of January, for instance, is "International Quality of Life Month." What better way to enhance your quality of life than getting a massage? January 15th is "Customer Service Day"; January 30th to 31st is "Ladies Bliss Days." Right there are three golden marketing opportunities in a month that is traditionally slow—people usually go overboard spending during the holidays, and January is often a month of people coming in redeeming gift certificates they received for Christmas, which may mean a lot of people but little cash flow.

There are so many holidays of appreciation for different populations. April has National Volunteer Week. May has Nurse's Week, Teacher's Week, and Police Officer's Week. Consider offering a discount to those people during their special week. There are so many opportunities for special promotions. If you follow the SBA's adage of performing a marketing activity every day, these are just a few examples of days you could come up with promotions for.

Carmen's Story

My Story

I do a lot of marketing based on "Appreciation Week." These exist throughout the year for different groups: Nurse's Appreciation Week, Teacher's Appreciation Week, Fireman's Appreciation Week, and so forth. Instead of expensive newspaper ads, I use my fax machine to publicize these. I just print a flyer on my computer offering $10 off on their first massage and fax it to the fire departments, the schools, or whomever I am targeting, and it always gets results—and I haven't spent any money to advertise it.

Holidays are only one consideration when developing your marketing calendar. If you have decided on a monthly amount you can spend, the next step is deciding what venues are going to be the most effective for you. One that you should not do without is the Yellow Pages. Consumers turn to the Yellow Pages every day when looking for goods and services. While your regulars may not need to look up your number, new clients, tourists, visitors from out of town, and so forth will go to the Yellow Pages looking for massage therapists. Small listings start as low as $35 per month in my small town—so for less than the price of one massage, I really can't afford not to have a listing.

In my town and in most places, local newspapers are usually expensive when it comes to display ads, so you want to get the most for your money. I have found through trial and error that one of the best times for newspaper advertising is when the paper prints a "magazine" issue—supplements to the regular paper that people tend to pull out and leave around long after the paper itself has gone into the trash. Some of the examples here in my town are a Bridal Issue, a Health and Fitness Issue, and the annual Fact Book, which is all about our county, the history of it, facts such as population, weather, listings of schools and churches, and business listings. The advertising department of the newspaper usually has these issues planned months in advance. In January, they are able to tell me what the magazine issues are going to be for the entire year, and that way I can pick and choose the ones I think I need to be advertised in, put it on my calendar, and plan ahead for spending that money.

Our county has a website that lists among other things (including a link to my website; more about that later in Chapter 22) the festivals and big events that are going to take place during the coming year. That allows me to plan for happenings that I want to participate in, and that goes on my marketing calendar as well. Other community service events that I normally plan or participate in go on my calendar as soon as I know about them. For instance, I have worked many times with a local hospital that holds health screenings in various venues throughout the year. They have held it right at my office several times in the past. In January, I can call the community health coordinator, and she can tell me most of the health events that are scheduled for the year. That way, I can go ahead and put those on my calendar as events that I want to participate in. The other great benefit to this is that the hospital pays to advertise that event. Besides the newspaper ads they place, it's mentioned on the radio and the local television station as a public service announcement, and on the day of the event the hospital brings a big sandwich sign and places it on the sidewalk right outside our door to attract passersby. It's an opportunity to get more exposure that I don't have to pay a cent for.

Since my goal is for my advertising budget and my marketing calendar to coexist in peaceful and profitable harmony, I need to take an accounting at the beginning of each year in order to be able to plan ahead and maximize my exposure while minimizing my cost. This year, I budgeted $5,000 for advertising. I already know how much my Yellow Pages ad costs, and the cost of advertising in the local newspaper's magazine issues I will want to participate in. After I deduct those items from my $5,000 total, I'll be left with approximately $2,400, so that means I can spend $200 per month and still stick to my budget for the coming year.

On my marketing calendar, I make a daily notation of what marketing activity I have done that day; whether it's just calling old clients I haven't seen lately, performing a community service duty, paid advertising or whatever. Whenever a new client comes in, I ask where they heard about us and track those results. At the end of the year, I can look back and see what worked and what didn't, and know what changes in strategy I need to make for the following year.

Appendix V lists holidays—the silly, the obscure, and the legitimate— for every day of the year. These were culled from a number of websites devoted to the subject. Websites are often ephemeral and disagree with each other, but since very few of the holidays listed are anything official, don't let it be a concern. Those days that I couldn't locate a holiday for, have a "Day in History" instead; something you could easily build a whole calendar around. Just as I mentioned Alexander Hamilton earlier, you could have an entire calendar marking the birthdays of famous people.

There are a lot of ways to be creative with the silly holidays. If you're fortunate enough to have one of those signs by the roadside, just putting a silly holiday on it daily or weekly will make people laugh and talk about it. Build promotions around them and list them in your newsletter or your e-mails and faxes to clients. You can combine a discount on massage with a donation to charity, for instance. April 13th is International Plant Appreciation Day. Announce that people bringing in a houseplant will get a 10% discount that day—and take the plants to a local nursing home at the end of the day. June 6th is Hunger Awareness Day. Offer a discount to anyone who brings in six canned items and give the food collected to the homeless

The Balanced Body

This is National Cow Appreciation Week. Bring your cow by our office and we'll give you $10 off on your massage!

shelter or local food bank. September 9th is Teddy Bear Day. Collect teddy bears for the children's hospital. There's no end to what you can come up with.

Your calendar is a marketing bonanza—but only if you utilize it. Remember: *don't let a day go by without performing a marketing activity.*

My Personal Journey

This Week's Activity: Creating My Marketing Calendar Date ____________________

For this week's activity, create your own marketing calendar. Utilize the silly holidays in Appendix V, appreciation days for special groups of people, famous birthdays, religious holidays, or whatever you like. Remember that your marketing calendar is meant to work in conjunction with your budget from Chapter 2, so you market yourself as cheaply as possible and make the best use of your advertising dollars.

My Goals

What's in my way?

What action can I take to remedy the situation?

One-Year Progress Update Date ____________________

POSITIVE AFFIRMATION: **Promoting myself is second nature to me.**

PART 2

Preparing for Your Trip

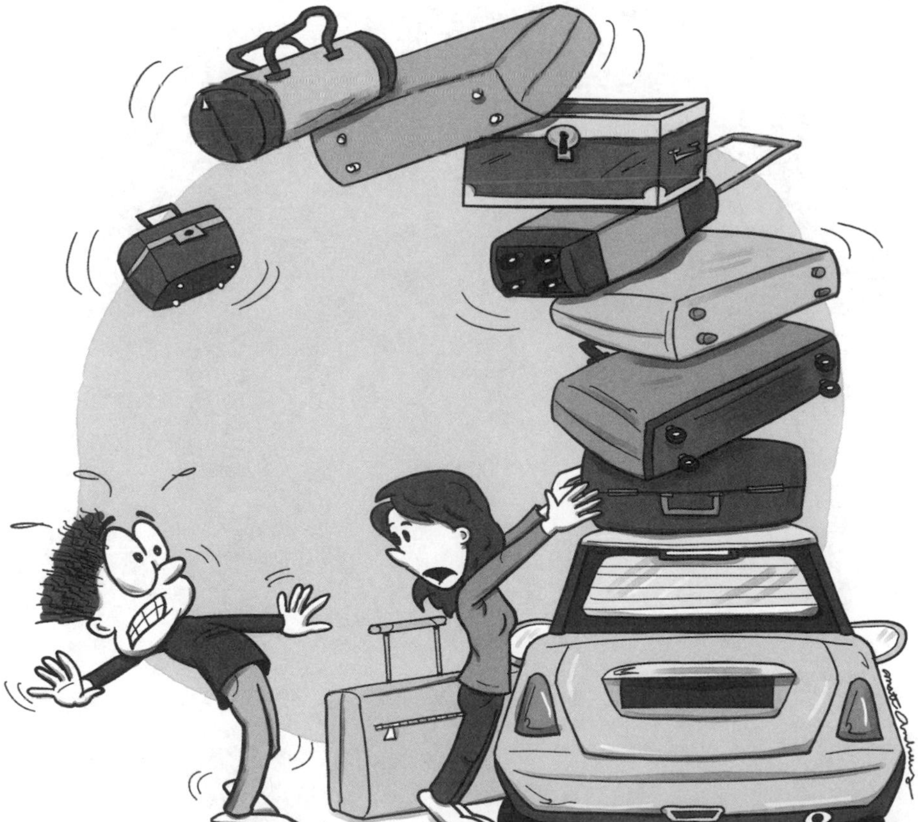

"I WANT TO MAKE SURE I HAVE ENOUGH CLOTHES FOR THE TRIP!"

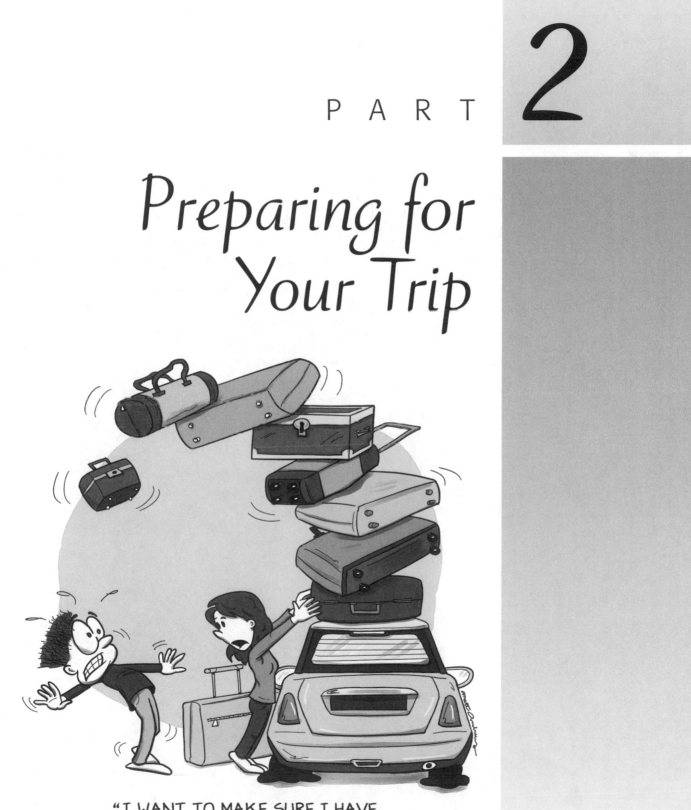

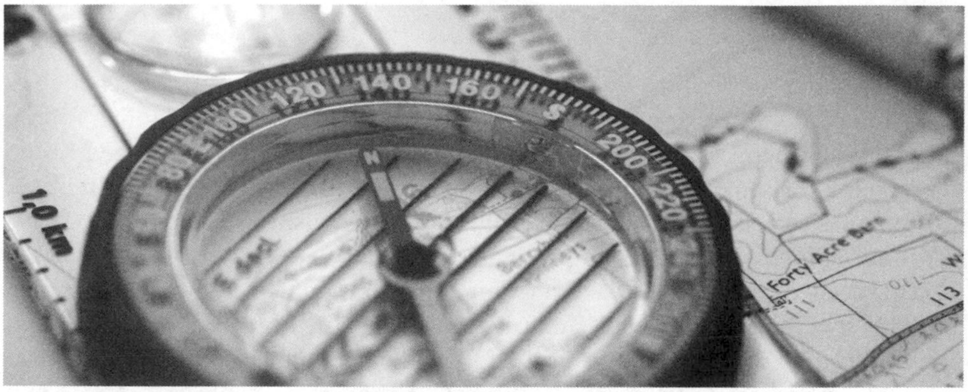

CHAPTER

4

Choosing a Name for Your Business

The person who makes a success of living is the one who sees his goal steadily and aims for it unswervingly. That is dedication.

—Cecil B. DeMille

What do you want the name of your business to convey about you and your services? That should be your primary consideration when choosing a name for your business.

Something like *Main Street Massage* is straightforward enough. It lets people know you're located on Main Street and you do massage—but not much else. That's not meant as a criticism; in a small town where everyone knows you, it may be enough. On the other hand, *Main Street Neuromuscular Therapy* gives the impression that you are a medically oriented massage therapist who is in business to get people out of pain.

Some therapists have fun with their business names by using puns or other plays on words, such as *Kneading Touch* or *Here's the Rub*. You won't become known for medical massage if your business name is *Here's the Rub*, but maybe you don't want to. If relaxation massage is your forte, *Here's the Rub* may be an okay name for your enterprise.

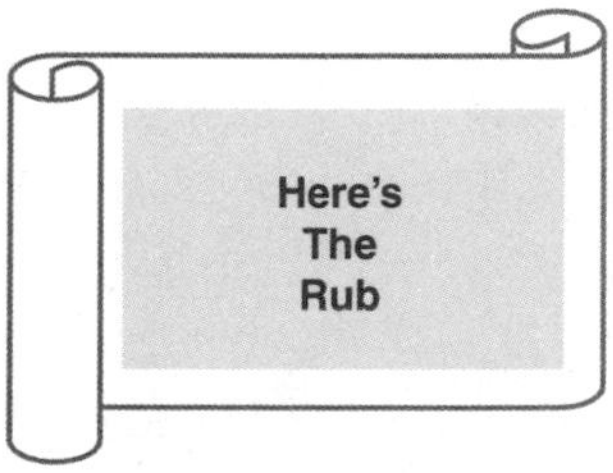

While there is something to be said for originality, some therapists have chosen obscure names that may be of personal meaning to them but that in reality are poor choices because the general public isn't familiar with the word or term. An example is *The Namaste Center.* One translation of *Namaste* is, "The God that lives in me honors the God that lives in you." People who haven't studied Indian mysticism probably don't know that. Another example is *Kookuburra Kare* (yes, I have actually seen both these names on massage businesses). Is it a day-care center, a rest home for elderly people, or a rehabilitation farm for Australian birds? Who knows? It doesn't say anything about massage and bodywork. If you should choose some obscure word or phrase for your business because it has a special personal meaning to you, then please put *Massage & Bodywork* as part of the name. The shorter and simpler it is, the easier it is for people to remember.

Your name is one of the first impressions people get of your business and may be a factor in whether or not they choose you when they're perusing the Yellow Pages. Of all the names mentioned above, if a newcomer in town looked in the phone book for someone who could treat their sciatica or carpal tunnel syndrome through massage, they would undoubtedly choose the business named *Main Street Neuromuscular Therapy.*

Speaking of the Yellow Pages, another consideration with your business name is *placement* in the phone book and other business directories. *Associated Massage Therapists* is going to be near the top of the list, while *Massage Associates* would be nearer the bottom. Another pitfall is choosing a name that's too long, such as *Associated Medical Massage Therapists & Bodywork Practitioners.* It won't fit well on a business card, and people just plain won't remember something that long.

You may choose to be known by your name. *Laura Allen, Licensed Massage Therapist*, isn't very exciting but it conveys what I do, if not how I do it. If you choose to go that route, you might want to put another line underneath for clarification, such as *Neuromuscular Therapy*, *Specializing in Pregnancy Massage* or *Swedish Massage.*

There are only so many names to go around. While traveling around teaching classes, I have seen at least fifty places named *Healing Touch* and another fifty named *Healing Hands.* If you are just going into business, it is wise to perform a name search or to have an attorney perform one for you, in order to avoid using a trademarked name or a name that is taken by other businesses, even if it isn't trademarked. In some states, particularly if you are incorporating, you will be obligated to do so; some state governments will do it for you if you provide them with the name you potentially want to use. If you're in a relatively small town, you should avoid choosing a name that sounds too close to another's business. If there's already a massage therapy business named *Healing Touch* in your town, then calling yours *Healing Hands* is not very original and is likely to confuse the public. It's easy to see how a new client that had an appointment at one would mistakenly show up at the other.

Even the *look* of your name on your signage, business cards, and other printed materials can give people a strong impression of your business. Consider these two examples:

The Spa **The Spa**

Which one of these names conjures up an image of a sleek, modern place and which one conjures up an image of a more traditional place, like a spa in an old-money country club? It's obvious.

If you are new to the business, consider making a short list of names that you like and then asking friends and family which name they think is the most appealing. If you've been in business for a long time, and feel that your name is well known, you probably don't want to change that. But if you're feeling stagnated in your practice, you might want to consider a name change—perhaps in conjunction with other changes you're going to make over the next year during your mission to revitalize your practice. You could move to a better location, have a nicer sign, or just redecorate your office and spruce up your menu of services.

If you've chosen your name and you're satisfied with it, it is now time to go forth and spread it around!

Jesse's Story

My Story

When I graduated from massage school, I went to work at a place called *Kneading Hands*. Even though the business had been established for over a year, almost daily we would get a call from someone thinking it was a bakery. When I went out on my own I chose the name Abbeville Therapeutic Massage. While it may not be a catchy play on words, no one is going to mistake me for the donut lady, either.

My Personal Journey

This Week's Activity: Choosing a Name for My Business Date ____________________

For this week's activity, choose some possible names for your business. Even if you plan to work for someone else, do this activity as an exercise in discerning names that are catchy and effective at conveying your intent as a bodyworker who wants a name that will contribute to the success of your business. After you choose some possible names, ask friends and family to help you choose the one that is best for your business.

My Goals

____

____

____

What's in my way?

____

____

____

What action can I take to remedy the situation?

____

____

____

One-Year Progress Update Date ____________________

____

____

____

POSITIVE AFFIRMATION: **My name is synonymous with success.**

CHAPTER

5

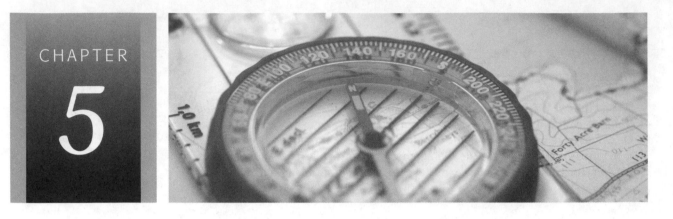

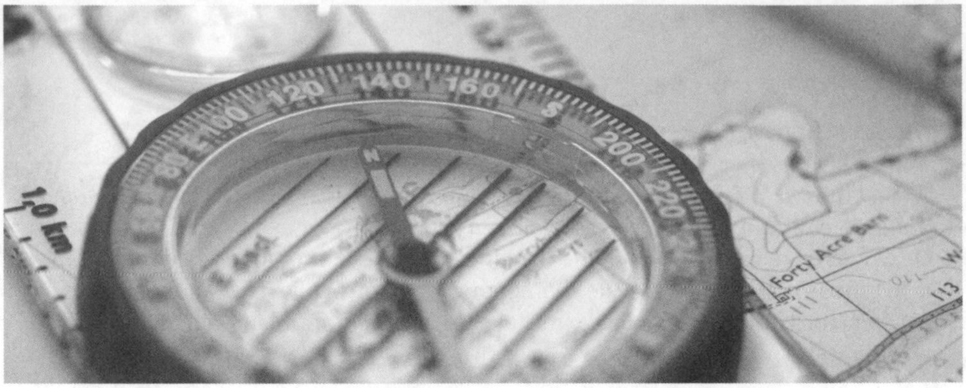

Making Your Product Stand Out From the Crowd

Action is the foundational key to all success.

—Tony Robbins

Hopefully by now you have realized that *you are the product*. Perhaps you have limited your practice to a specific modality—you only want to do pregnancy massage or craniosacral massage. There's a niche for you. Whether you do Swedish massage or you are a multi-skilled therapist who uses the eclectic approach, you can still make yourself stand out from the crowd. Create something—a signature—something you're known for service-wise, that will make people think you're a cut above the rest.

My Story

Suzanne's Story

I just love gadgets and trying new things. There are so many products out there made for massage therapy—various implements like the rubber balls, magnets, vibrators, chi machines, steamers and the like, and something new being invented all the time. I have a passion for collecting these, and my clients love them! I have a shelf in my massage room with all my tools on it, and new people always want to know what things are. I just ask if they'd like to try something new, and almost everybody does. I can put my chi machine on the foot of the massage table and just hold a client's head for a few minutes, or use the massage bongers on their back, and they feel great. My regular clients are always asking me what my latest toy is, and they look forward to trying it out, whatever it is. I think it makes me stand out from the crowd.

A male therapist I know who's in his 70s and still doing massage every day always ends the massage by having you relax with a hot towel placed on your face for a few minutes. It opens your sinuses, of course, if you've been lying prone, but more than that it just feels *nice*. It's a little extra that costs him nothing, but I have heard the compliments from others who have been to him—"Oh, Bob always gives you a nice hot towel at the end." People love it. Another therapist I sometimes visit offers everyone their choice of an herbal eye pillow or chamomile tea bags to put on their eyes while they're supine. Another acquaintance purchases beautifully printed cards with positive affirmations on them as a give-away to her clients. Every client who enters the treatment room at her establishment finds one of these cards on the massage table. The therapist tells me that many times the client will say to her, "That's exactly what I needed to hear today." Those little treats only take a minute and are minimal in cost, but they make the total experience of the massage just a little nicer—and that's enough to make people keep coming back.

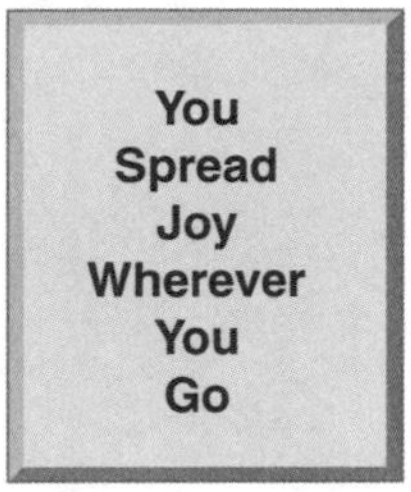
You
Spread
Joy
Wherever
You
Go

If you *are* limiting your practice to a specialty, (i) it helps if there's a demand for your service, and (ii) you can *create that demand* yourself. Pregnancy massage, for instance, is not hard to market because there are pregnant women almost everywhere at any given time. But if you live in a small town or rural area, the local populace may not know what craniosacral is, or the benefits of it, so give some free demonstrations. Generate interest by talking about it whenever and wherever you have the opportunity. Be prepared with your "elevator speech" (more about that in Chapter 6), to tell people the high points of your work in a couple of minutes in such an interesting way, they'll feel like they'll be missing out if they don't give it a try.

Unless you are filling a really unique niche or the lone massage therapist in a rural area, it's highly likely that there's plenty of competition. People have a choice about where to go; they need a good reason to come to *you*. If you're new to the trade and looking for your first job, that employer needs a good reason to hire you instead of the next therapist just out of massage school. You can stack the deck in your favor by observing one rule: *presentation is everything*.

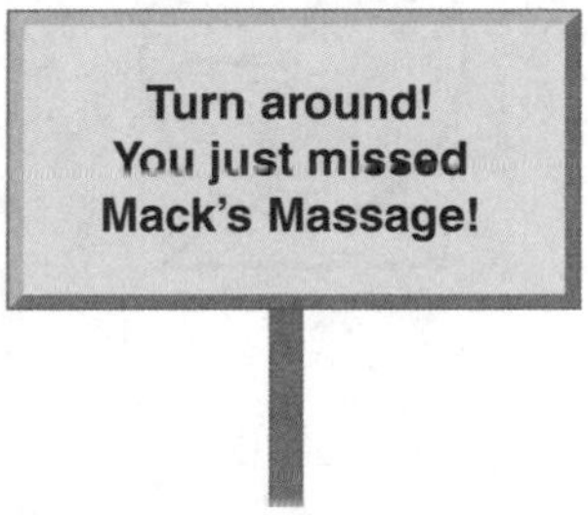
Turn around!
You just missed
Mack's Massage!

Presentation Is Everything

If you are just out of school and seeking employment in someone else's establishment, dress professionally when you go looking for a job. While there are a few massage schools that require students to wear whites or scrubs, many have no dress code. During my traveling to different schools teaching continuing education classes, I've seen many students in sweats, cut-off jeans, holey t-shirts with beer advertisements on them, revealing clothing, and barefooted in class. Your school may have been casual about it, but don't let that attitude carry over into the job market. Dress as if you are going to a business meeting. You are, and the subject under scrutiny is *you.*

A professional massage therapist is a member of the health care team. When you go to the doctor, she's usually dressed in business attire and a white lab coat. That looks professional, and inspires confidence. What if you showed up for an appointment with a physician, and she was barefoot, wearing ripped jeans and a Grateful Dead tank top; would you feel the same about her abilities and professionalism? You don't have to wear a three-piece suit to interviews or to work, but do be conscious of what image you are projecting with your clothes.

I'm all for freedom of expression and exercising personal taste, but you must realize that the way you present yourself is going to have an effect on the clientele you attract. If you want affluent business people for clients, or you plan to focus on geriatric massage, you should avoid wearing your hair in a purple buzz cut, multiple facial piercing, and shredded clothing. If you only want the Goth/Old Hippie crowd to come to your door, feel free to let your inner fashionista run wild, but bear in mind if you are job-hunting that visible tattoos, piercings, and dreadlocks will automatically remove you from the potential employee list of many places, regardless of how talented a massage therapist you are. It may not be fair, but it's true.

When you're trying to attract clientele, in addition to giving a good presentation of yourself, take a critical look at your workspace as well. Whether you own your own place or work for someone else, an office and/or massage room that is spotlessly clean and clutter-free will inspire your clients' confidence in you and is a crucial part of your professional image. It doesn't mean you have to be the unpaid maid in someone else's establishment, but if you work there and it's dirty or messy, it reflects upon you.

Be on Time

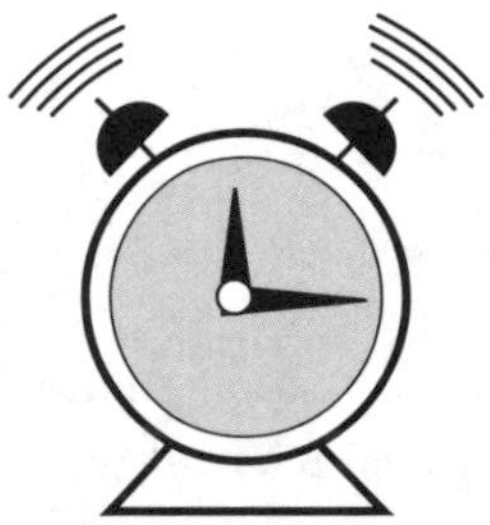

There should actually be five P's of marketing: Punctuality is probably the number one complaint of the American public when they have a doctor's appointment or are expecting the plumber at their house. Nearly everyone has experienced waiting for someone like that long past your appointed time. It's irritating, and you get the feeling that your time isn't viewed with the same importance as theirs. Time is money to you, and time is money to the client. She may be taking her lunch hour to get an appointment with you, or fitting you in between two business appointments. Start on time, every time. Clients who arrive on time for their appointment should not have to sit and wait for you to finish up with the last person, collect their money and reschedule them, change your table, use the bathroom, wash your hands, get a drink of water, answer the phone, and so forth. They should be able to feel confident that their nine o'clock appointment is really going to start at nine o'clock, not nine twenty-five.

A word to the wise: if you're on time, but your client isn't, this is one of those times when you have to follow your schedule and your conscience. If your client arrives late, and you have other clients scheduled after her, you have to politely say, "Ma'am, I'm afraid we still have to end your appointment at one. I have someone scheduled behind you." Of course, if you don't have another appointment, it is entirely up to you whether or not to give her the whole hour. In my busy office, the clock starts ticking when their appointment is scheduled, and stops at the appointed time. And yes, they pay for the full hour, even if they were late and only got forty minutes. The therapist saved that hour for them, and they are expected to pay for it. It's one of our policies, and no one has ever complained about it. It's something you'll have to decide for yourself how to handle.

Communication Skills

One of the most important parts of your personal presentation is your ability to communicate with and listen to the client effectively. Give them your undivided attention and focus on what they are saying, especially during the intake process. Let them feel that during their appointment time, *it is all about them*; after all, it is. They are paying for your time and attention. Give it to them. Some people prefer silence during their massage, and others want to talk; they want someone to listen to them. Don't offer unqualified advice—just listen. Reading body language is a key skill of a professional massage therapist, as some people will hesitate to tell you the pressure is too deep, or they'd like more, from shyness or for fear of hurting your feelings. Be grounded, centered, and constantly tuned in to the comfort level of the client.

In the same vein, the burden of effective communication is on *you*. As massage therapists, we are educated to the fact that the place where pain is may not necessarily be where the problem lies. The public, in general, is not educated about referred pain unless their physician has explained it to them. You need to tell the client, for instance, why your work is focusing on the side opposite their pain—that the muscles on one side have become shortened, and the other side is trying to compensate. Otherwise, they may have the feeling that you didn't pay attention to their needs.

Years ago, before I became a therapist, I recall leaving a massage and crying from pain and frustration on the way home. I had gone to a therapist I didn't know well, and I was in pain. I told her the reason I was there was because I had this awful pain in my right hip. She worked me over good—everywhere except where I had told her I needed it. I was hurting just as bad when I left her office as I had been when I walked in the door and I was frustrated as well. I never went back to her.

A Positive Attitude

A positive attitude is a given. You don't want to visit a therapist who greets you unenthusiastically, complains about the weather or lack of business, or how tired she is. You want to visit someone who acts happy to see you, and who is grateful that out of all the therapists in town, you chose her. That's exactly what your clients want too.

If you are interviewing for a job, your attitude, above all else, is probably either the deal-breaker or the reason you'll get the job. Employers like enthusiasm. They want to know that you'll make their clients feel welcome. During the interview, don't complain about your last job—or anything else. If you're just out of school and hoping to land your first job, stress your strong points without bragging, in a straightforward manner, such as, "I really enjoy performing the spa techniques I learned in school, and that's why I want to work here at the Mountain Breeze Spa. I've been trained in mud wraps, scrubs, and paraffin treatments, and of course I'll be glad to learn the other treatments your spa offers." What you lack in experience can be made up for with enthusiasm and presentation.

Whether you are seeking employment or going into business on your own, put yourself in the place of the interviewer or the customer. Dressing professionally, cultivating good communication skills, giving the client your full attention, displaying a smile and a positive attitude, punctuality, a clean office—those are the characteristics that will make you stand out above the crowd, and are just as important as your ability to give a good massage.

My Personal Journey

This Week's Activity: Making My Product Stand Out from the Crowd Date ______________

For this week's activity, brainstorm for ideas that will make you stand out among other massage therapists. What services you can offer; what benefits your clients can receive by coming to you instead of going elsewhere; what special touches you are going to give that will make *you* the massage therapist of choice.

My Goals

____

____

____

What's in my way?

____

____

____

What action can I take to remedy the situation?

____

____

____

One-Year Progress Update Date ______________

____

____

____

POSITIVE AFFIRMATION: **I am a superior product that must be marketed as such.**

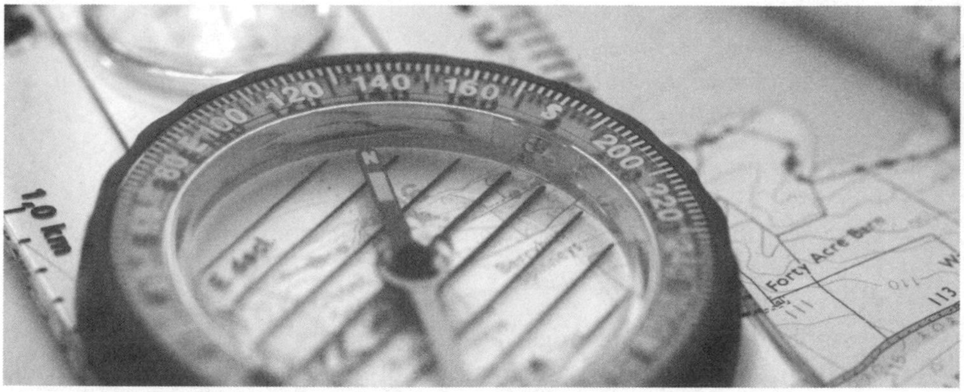

CHAPTER 6

Your Elevator Speech

An elevator speech is a prepared script that you can give in three minutes or less to tell people what you do and how it can be of benefit to them. Can you give a good three-minute speech about massage in general, and specifically about your business? Unless you stay home and live like a hermit, chances are you have many opportunities during the day when you could give an elevator speech that will make an impression on people. If you don't already have a prepared elevator speech, now is the time to cultivate that. Practice with your family or standing in front of a mirror until it becomes second nature.

I use my elevator speech a lot. Say I'm in the grocery store and the person in line behind me has their arm in a cast. People aren't usually offended when you ask what happened; most will readily tell you. There's the opportunity to hand them a card and say, "When that cast comes off, massage therapy can really help you regain your strength and mobility in that arm. I'm Laura Allen and my massage therapy office is on South Main Street. Please give me a call." That took less than a minute and it's enough—unless they say, "Really? I've never had a massage. How can it help?" Then the *real* elevator speech can begin. "Massage increases circulation. Just getting fresh blood and oxygen to the injured area will help your recovery. For injury rehabilitation in a case like yours, we'll do some gentle joint mobilizations to help you get the flexibility back and to strengthen your muscles again, which tend to lose some tone when they're immobilized in a cast. Massage really soothes the pain when you're recovering, too."

New Clients Just Ahead

That's only one scenario. There's the stressed-out mother you see shopping with three kids in tow, the pregnant waitress at your favorite restaurant, your mailman who you notice is limping recently as if his sciatica is acting up, your arthritic great-aunt; the list goes on and on. You may think you don't know that many people, when in reality, there are dozens of people that you have contact with. You have to start thinking of everyone you meet as a potential client—and why shouldn't they be?

My Story

Cora's Story

I am a shy person and I was initially nervous talking to people about the benefits of massage, but it didn't take me long to find out that people are truly interested. The more I talked about it the more comfortable I became, to the point where I have even gone and spoken to groups about it. Talking about massage educates people and it has helped me to become a more social person.

We all learn the benefits of massage in the early days of massage school. To refresh your memory, here are just a few things you can say about massage. It:

- Increases circulation of blood and lymph.
- Increases joint mobility and flexibility.
- Lengthens the shortened muscles and frees adhesions that cause pain.
- Is a great antidote to stress.
- Can reduce anxiety.
- Eases the discomforts of pregnancy.
- Can help such conditions as carpal tunnel syndrome, sciatica, back pain, TMJ syndrome, fibromyalgia, arthritis, bursitis (you keep going, you know the list is long, and they may have already said, "I have so-and-so, can massage help that?).
- Can help speed recovery after an injury.

Then, you'll need some one-liners that describe *your* practice, such as:

- Hi, I'm Laura Allen and I'm a licensed massage therapist.
- My office is conveniently located on Main Street.
- I accept insurance.
- I'm open Monday through Saturday from nine to six.
- I specialize in (injury recovery, pregnancy massage, whatever).
- I do house calls.
- I get a lot of doctor referrals; I can give you references (this one works really well).
- I give a discount to senior citizens.
- I sell gift certificates.
- I offer package deals.

Those are just a few of the kind of things you should say in your elevator speech. Be friendly without being pushy, and always have a card in your hand ready to give them as you're talking. Your goal is not to "make a sale," but to create a conversation that will make the listener feel as if you are there to help them solve a problem that they have.

Don't change your demeanor when you're giving your elevator speech. You don't have to sound like an overenthusiastic cheerleader; you just need to sound like yourself and sound genuine. Every listener is a potential client, but you're more apt to get them as a client if you treat them like a person instead of a source of revenue. If you have the time and they want to tell you in detail about their injury, listen. People feel important when someone listens to them, and you want everyone who comes to you to feel important *because you have made them feel that way.* If you can manage to make someone feel important during your elevator speech, just think of what you'll do for them when they come in for their actual appointment!

My Personal Journey

This Week's Activity: Developing My Elevator Speech Date ____________________

For this week's activity, you are going to develop your elevator speech and practice the delivery. It will be helpful if you write a script—what you want to say about massage and yourself—and practice giving it to friends and family until you have it down pat.

My Goals

___

___

___

What's in my way?

___

___

___

What action can I take to remedy the situation?

___

___

___

One-Year Progress Update Date ____________________

___

___

___

POSITIVE AFFIRMATION: **I am a great communicator.**

CHAPTER

7

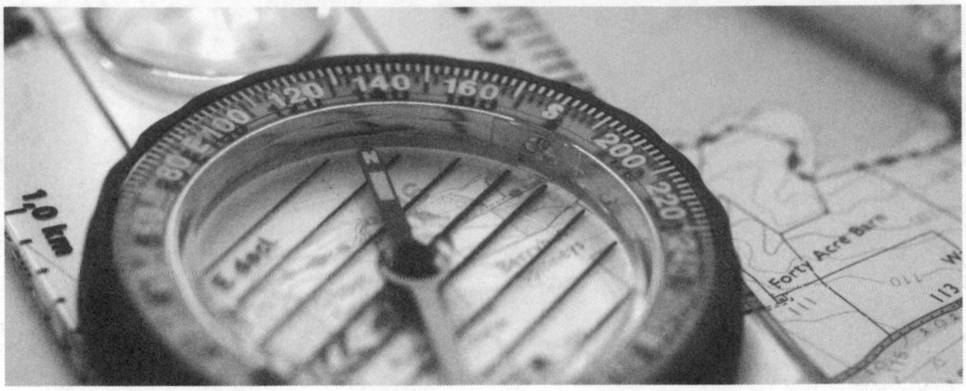

Your Business Literature

Believe in yourself! Have faith in your abilities! Without a humble but reasonable confidence in your own powers you cannot be successful or happy.

—Norman Vincent Peale

Your business literature includes your business cards, brochures, menus of services, letterheads, invoices, receipts, intake forms, welcome-to-the-practice postcards, and any other imprinted paper products that you give to customers. Think of everything with your name and/or your company name on it as marketing material.

You may make your own on your computer, purchase them ready-made from one of the companies that cater to the massage trade, or have custom designs created and printed by a professional graphic designer or printing company. Whichever way you choose to go, there are several points to consider that can have a big impact on your professional image.

Does it make sense to have green and black business cards along with pink and purple brochures? No, it doesn't. If you are going the cheaper route for now and printing your own on your personal computer, you can still have a professional look by using good business paper stock and having *continuity* with your marketing materials—brochure paper that matches your business cards looks much more professional than materials that are mismatched.

Find a font that you like and use it for all printed materials. When choosing a font for printed materials, think about what you are trying to convey about your business. If you decide to use an unusual font for your name, beware of using it throughout the rest of the literature. For the meat-and-potatoes information you are trying to give, use a font that is simple and easy to read. You don't want people to struggle through reading your brochure.

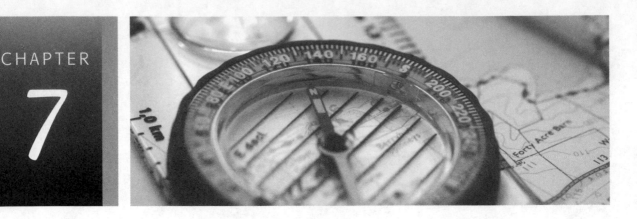

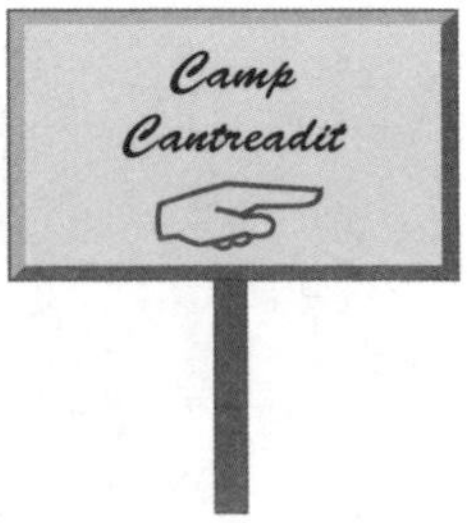

Whether you are printing your own or hire a professional, be sure to proofread *and* use the spell checker function. The spell checker doesn't differentiate between *suite* and *sweet*; they're both spelled correctly, and if they are misused the spell checker doesn't catch it. Professional designers and printers are not immune from making typos or transposing numbers. You should be provided with a proof prior to the final product being printed. Read it carefully yourself and ask a few other people to read it—customers, family, whoever is around. In addition to looking for mistakes, ask for feedback. Is the printed product attractive and easy to read? Avoid light colored fonts on dark backgrounds. They're too hard to read.

Leave a little white space. A card or brochure that has so much text and/or so many graphics that there's no space is distracting rather than informative. Strive for a clean uncluttered look, regardless of the theme you choose to use. Remember, the goal for your business literature is to provide information to the client in a way that is appealing and easy to understand.

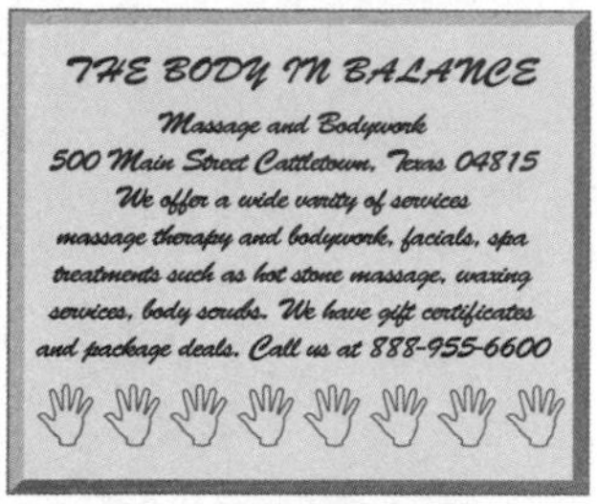

More about business cards: they're useless unless you have them with you. Many is the time I've met someone, another therapist I might want to network with, or a tradesman of some sort who's services I may be in need of, and they say, "I don't have any cards with me, let me write it down on this scrap of paper." That is *so* unprofessional. You should have a supply of business cards with you at all times to give to people you've just met or haven't seen in a long time. Keep extras in your car. Go to your closet and put a few into the pockets of each of your jackets, coats, and sweaters. If you switch purses frequently, get an inexpensive card case and fill it for each one—that way, you won't be caught without.

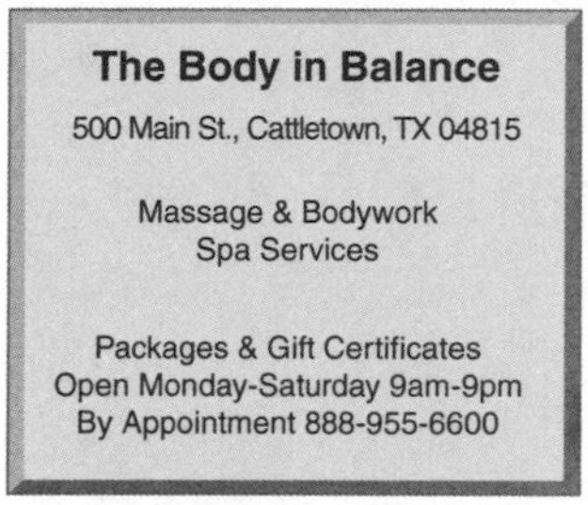

Kay's Story

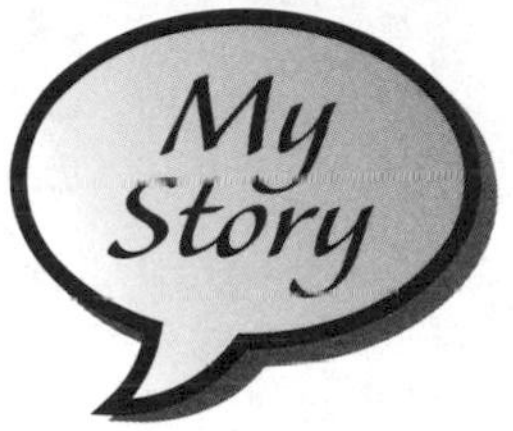

I give a business card to every single person I meet—the checker at the grocery store, people I do business with, waitresses, everybody. Sometimes they call the next day, but many times someone will call and say, "I met you last year at Susan's party . . ." and they're just now getting around to calling. They kept the card for months or even a couple of years sometimes before coming in—proof to me that giving away cards is never a wasted effort.

Do you give one to everybody you meet? If the answer is no, the next question is *why not*? When leaving a tip in a restaurant, leave a business card, too. When paying a bill at a local business, put a card in the envelope with your check. Each time someone gives you their business card, give them one of yours. Better yet, don't wait for them to give you one of theirs—give them yours first! Many restaurants, shopping centers, and so forth have racks or bulletin boards where you can put your cards. Take advantage of every one you come across. It doesn't matter if it's not right in your neighborhood. The therapists in my office have clients that come from many miles away. Maybe there's not a therapist in their neighborhood, or they've moved away and just prefer to make the trip back to see the therapist they're comfortable with instead of looking for someone new.

Be sure that physicians, chiropractors, and other health professionals that you have a mutual referral relationship with have a supply of your cards on hand (and that you have theirs as well). It's nice for you to supply your own card holder—just a plain plastic one. All the therapists in my office have individual cards, and they're all on the front desk in matching plastic holders. A new person joined the staff once, and brought in a very fancy polished marble card holder that was four inches taller than everyone else's, and I wouldn't let him use it. It gave an impression of somehow being superior to the others.

Don't forget about your customers. Always give them an extra card or two to share with others. If you are not marketing yourself in this simplest of ways, now is the time to start.

Brochures serve a variety of purposes. You'll need a brochure of your own that details your contact information, your operating hours, menu of services if it will fit on the same brochure, and your pricing structure. Other pertinent information, such as whether or not you accept insurance or do house calls, should also be part of the brochure. In addition to our office brochure, I also purchase brochures from a massage supply company, because they're informative to the clients. Some of the ones I have are *Chiropractic: A Compliment to Massage; Your First Massage; The Benefits of Massage; Sports and Massage; Pregnancy and Massage;* and so forth. These cost anywhere from ten to fifty cents each, but they're invaluable for educating your clients, and in the long run save you time you might have spent answering questions. Our office brochure is put in the envelope with every gift certificate sold.

It's a good idea to visit local gyms, salons, realty offices, community centers, and other places that will allow you to display your business cards and brochures. I reciprocate at my office by having one shelf that is devoted to displaying cards for other local business people. If a new person asks me if they may leave their cards or brochures, I ask them if they will take some of mine in return and the answer is nearly always yes. You can't be everywhere at once. Good quality, professional cards and brochures can spread your good name—as long as *you* spread them around. Don't forget to check back periodically to refresh the supply.

You are using your business cards, brochures, and other printed materials to represent your business. If there are other massage businesses in close proximity to yours, try to avoid using the same look on your literature that they have on theirs. This may seem like a small thing, but it can have an impact on your business. I order my own business cards from a company that caters to our trade. Last weekend while teaching at a massage school about a hundred and fifty miles from my home, I noticed that the owner has the same business cards that I have. That's okay, but if she was located across the street from me, I would want to be sure mine was different from hers.

It's a nice touch on brochures, invoices, and receipts to have the line "Thank you for patronizing our business" or something similar—just an extra bit of customer appreciation.

My Personal Journey

This Week's Activity: Developing Professional Business Literature Date ____________________

For this week's activity, begin creating your professional business literature, starting with your business cards. If you are still a student, you could make cards that say "Student Massage Therapist." Be sure that you are in compliance with your state laws, if there are any, governing the wording of your cards. You may want to create a logo for yourself, or enroll the help of a graphics designer who might trade their skills in exchange for massage. Look through your business textbook for forms you may want to personalize to fit your situation and adapt them as needed.

My Goals

____

____

____

What's in my way?

____

____

____

What action can I take to remedy the situation?

____

____

____

One-Year Progress Update Date ____________________

____

____

____

POSITIVE AFFIRMATION: **My business literature reflects my professionalism.**

CHAPTER

8

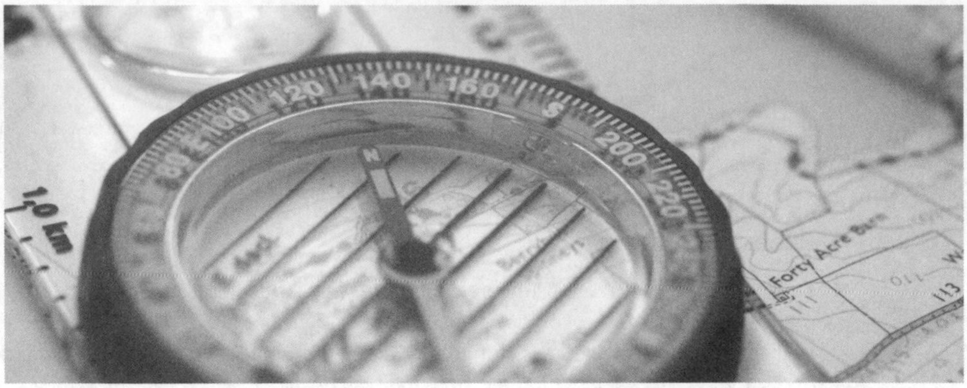

Your Menu of Services

Success is to be measured not so much by the position that one has reached in life but by the obstacles he has overcome.

—Booker T. Washington

Your menu of services was briefly touched on in Chapter 7 along with other pieces of business literature. Let's talk about the meat and potatoes of your menu.

If you only practice one modality, you may think you don't need a menu of services. You're wrong! For instance, you're trained in Swedish massage and that's it. Believe it or not, you can dress that up and add a few things to make your menu look more varied and inviting. Offer shorter sessions or longer sessions. Think of all the variations of Swedish massage, such as sports massage—Swedish on overdrive—or pregnancy massage, which is basically just a Swedish massage with special attention paid to the contraindications of pregnancy and the needs of an expectant mother, such as propping up with pillows, and being sure she's lying in a comfortable position. Likewise, geriatric massage is primarily Swedish massage with a focus on the special considerations and contraindications of the elderly. Like the pregnant woman, an elder may need special propping with pillows and may be uncomfortable lying prone; deeper massage may need to be avoided because of osteoporosis or other complications. Sports massage, though mainly derived from Swedish, has special protocols depending on whether the massage is performed pre-event, post-event, or while the athlete is in training. Be sure you know what you're doing, or you could adversely affect the competitive outcome of your client by performing the wrong massage. Don't perform sedative massage on someone who's about to run a marathon. There are at least several variations on Swedish massage you can mention on your menu.

In states that have licensure, or if you're maintaining AMTA membership or National Certification, you're obligated to take continuing education classes. If you've been practicing long enough to have attended continuing education classes, surely you've learned something else that you could add to your menu. There are also plenty of home study videos that will allow you to expand your skills and your menu of services.

If you are in an office with other practitioners, you could offer four-handed massage or couples massage. Your menu should make the treatments sound relaxing and enticing. Instead of just *Swedish Massage, $50 an hour*, say it like this:

> Swedish Massage, designed to relieve stress and muscle tension, guaranteed to make you float away on a cloud of relaxed bliss. One hour $50.

Which one of those massages would you rather have? I want the one that's going to make me float away on a cloud of relaxed bliss, don't you? That's *marketing!* If you specialize in medical massage, neuromuscular therapy, or other modalities directed at getting people out of pain, be sure your menu includes a listing of the conditions you specialize in, such as sciatica, fibromyalgia, or TMJ dysfunction. If you practice other modalities, list them all, along with their benefits and some other details about the technique, pricing, and length of session. For instance, lots of people don't know what Shiatsu is. Instead of *Shiatsu, $60 an hour*, say this:

> Shiatsu is a traditional Oriental therapy evolved from 5,000 years of healing arts. Shiatsu is normally performed with the client fully clothed on a floor mat or a table lowered close to the floor. Utilizing finger and palm pressure on different points of the body, Shiatsu can address many issues, particularly fatigue and stress. This is one of the most beneficial and relaxing massages you will ever have. One hour $60.

Doesn't that sound much more interesting?

A cheap and very profitable thing to add to your menu is paraffin for the hands and feet. You don't need any special skills to do it, and you can get started for very little money. It's an add-on service that can easily put an extra $10 or $20 onto the price of a session, and it doesn't take much time, either. You might want to allow an extra five or ten minutes for a massage appointment that includes a paraffin dip. Paraffin is so cheap, I can give a free dip to any one who comes in on their birthday, for instance. Heaven forbid, if anyone in the office is running behind and a client has to wait a few minutes, I give them a complimentary paraffin dip for having to wait. It doesn't even cost a quarter, and it spreads good will.

How about aromatherapy massage? Aromatherapy is an art and a science; if you've never attended a class, please don't indiscriminately put oils on people, because there are many contraindications. However, once you've educated yourself to those, just add a few oils to the massage and a few dollars to the price. You can even warm the plain oil you normally use for massage and call it *Hot Oil Massage* and charge $10 more for the massage.

Another cheap service is one I call the Peppermint Foot Rub. I rub the feet for about 20 minutes, basically a reflexology-type session using no oils or crème—giving the feet a good workout—followed by rubbing them briskly with peppermint essential oil and wrapping them in a hot towel for ten minutes. It's a shorter session, but people love it and it's booked frequently during lunch hour. Again, it doesn't require any special skills—you rub feet anyway—and the only added cost is a few drops of essential oils.

In addition to what services are available, your menu should also list the obvious—your address and phone number—but don't stop there. Your hours of operation, your cancellation policy, that you sell gift certificates, or offer outcalls should be on your menu as well. Your menu of services may be the only brochure you need if you can include all the pertinent information. If you have the space, you might solicit a couple of client testimonials to include. As mentioned in Chapter 7, be sure that they are professional looking, typo-free, descriptive, and easy to read.

Your menu of services is a great marketing tool. Always have a supply with you, just as you do your business cards.

My Story

Martha's Story

I have a plastic box attached to my front door that holds my menu of services. If people stop by after hours, or when I'm in with a client and have the outer door locked, they can take one. I also have a small notepad and pen attached to the door with instructions for people to drop their note in the mail slot if they would like to schedule an appointment, pick up a gift certificate, or just get information by return call. If you're a lone practitioner, as I am, this will help you get appointments you might otherwise have missed.

My Personal Journey

This Week's Activity: Creating My Menu of Services Date ______________

For this week's activity, create a menu of services; or if you are already a practitioner, look at revamping the one you already have in order to make it more attractive and expansive. Don't forget modalities you have learned in continuing education classes. Be sure it's easy to read and free of spelling and grammar mistakes.

My Goals

What's in my way?

What action can I take to remedy the situation?

One-Year Progress Update Date ______________

POSITIVE AFFIRMATION: **My menu of services showcases my practice in the best possible light.**

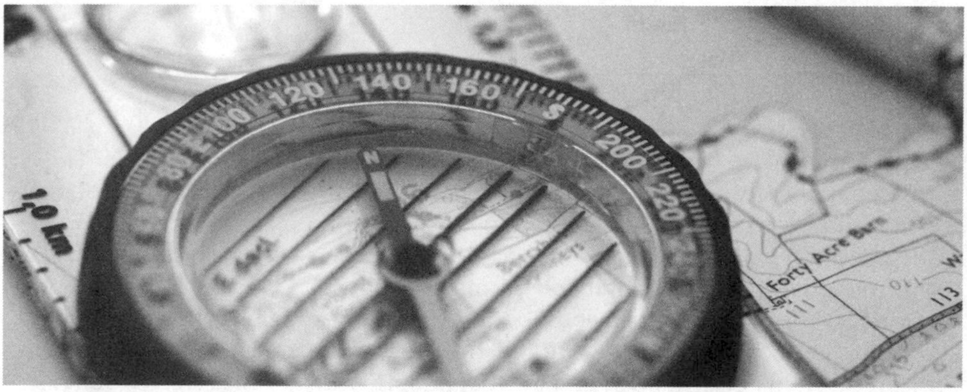

CHAPTER 9

Your Telephone

> *You are a product of your environment. So choose the environment that will best advance you toward your objective. Analyze your life in terms of its environment. Are the things around you helping you toward success, or are they holding you back?*
>
> —Clement Stone

Your telephone is a vital part of your business and your communications, and an important part of your professional image. Your telephone can be a powerful sales tool. As a total package with your answering machine and your fax machine, it can actually make or break your business.

Telephone Manners

Your telephone demeanor is often the first impression people have of you. Answering in a pleasant, business-like manner is a must. If someone other than yourself answers the phone in your office, adopt a uniform greeting and have everyone use it, like "Thanks for calling Main Street Massage; how can I help you?" or something similar. For those of you who practice from a home office, this should be of particular consideration to you. Consider having an extra line or getting an extra cell phone that is totally devoted to your business. It's a tax deduction, and this way you don't have to answer your home telephone with a business message, but you're still presenting a professional image. If you do practice at home, and you have a spouse, children, or teenagers who also answer the phone, you probably know from past experience it is easy to miss a business call—"Oh, yeah, Mom, some lady called three hours ago and wants a massage but I forgot to write down her name and number," and that's certainly not going to help you or the client. It's also hard to make your children answer the home phone as if it were a business tool. You don't want a client to call your home and get your 15-year-old son answering with, "Yo, whassup?"

My Story

Austin's Story

Guilty as charged! I choose to work from a home office so I can be near my young child, and being the proud parent I am, my answering machine message was recorded by my four-year-old son. I really thought it was cute, in spite of the fact that my son stuttered a little through the message and left a few silences that went on too long. I guess I was oblivious to the amount of hang-up calls I was getting until a client actually came out and told me she dreaded calling and getting the message. I had never stopped to think that people who don't have kids wouldn't think it was as cute as I do, or that the lengthy message was a turn-off. My feelings were a little hurt, but I swallowed that and thanked the client for letting me know. My message now sounds like a professional massage therapist recorded it—just like it should—and I don't get near as many hang-ups as I used to.

CAUTION

Don't try to be too cute on the phone. One therapist I know has a message during which she is giggling while recording the message. She sounds drunk, and I've told her that, to no avail. Another has her three-year-old leaving a barely intelligible message. She thinks it's cute; in reality it's very unprofessional sounding and I would personally hang up on it before leaving a message about trying to book a massage. Another one I know has very loud reggae music playing in the background. You can barely hear her speak on account of it, but she's oblivious to it and thinks it's a great-sounding message. She's in denial!

An Important Sales Tool

I have called massage therapists before, and have not gotten voicemail or an answering machine. Apparently those people have all the business they need. If you *don't* have all the business you need, you definitely need an answering machine or voicemail, and you should use your message as a selling tool. Just having, "This is Jim, leave a message," doesn't convey anything to anybody. This is better: "Thanks for calling Main Street Massage. I'm with a client right now, but I will return your call shortly if you will leave a message. The special this month is an hour of massage and a facial for $75." You've just given them something to think about while they wait for the return call. Check your messages frequently and return calls in a timely manner. If it's a first-time caller, be especially prompt in getting back to them. Even if you have to tell them you're all booked, let them know that quickly so they can look elsewhere.

If you have the feature on your phone that allows people to listen to music while they're on hold, get rid of that and replace it with a sales speech: "Thank you for waiting. Your call is important to us. We have a special on holiday gift certificates. Buy five and receive six, or buy ten and you'll receive twelve." Update your message regularly—at least each time the special offer changes.

It goes without saying that your phone number should be on every piece of business literature and advertising that you have. The Yellow Pages have been mentioned in several other chapters, but I will reinforce here that it's one piece of advertising you should definitely pay for. Just think of how many times you personally need a service person of some sort—where do you turn? That's right, the Yellow Pages.

If you can, get a phone number that's easy to remember, like (888)-MASSAGE.

Your Cell Phone

Let's assume you have a business phone *and* a cell phone. If you don't, you should. The thinking here is in line with the reasons mentioned above for having a separate line for your business. You can use your cell while you're away from your office to check your messages, or you can forward all office calls to your cell, with a special ring, so you'll know to answer the phone in a professional manner.

Broadcast Faxing

Broadcast faxing is a cheap way to spread the news about specials, events, and so forth for your business. As a member of the Chamber of Commerce, one of the benefits I have is the ability to broadcast fax to all the other Chamber members, a very substantial number of people. I don't even have to do it myself; I just fax the notice I want broadcast to the Chamber office, and they do it for me. You can of course collect fax numbers on your own; you might even have a space for it on your intake form along with the statement that they can provide it if they would like to be notified of specials and such by fax. Incidentally, the Chamber members here have a signed agreement to be notified by fax. Faxing people who don't agree to it is paramount to spam just like e-mail spam, so don't do it, or at the least, have a statement at the bottom to the effect that they may call or e-mail you if they don't wish to receive faxes from you. You can never err too much on the side of integrity in your business practices.

My Personal Journey

This Week's Activity: Telephone Marketing Date ______________

For this week's activity, you are going to improve the quality of your telephone marketing. Write a short script for the way you are going to answer your telephone. Write a list of frequently asked questions that potential clients have, and have a script ready to answer them quickly and efficiently. Change the message on your answering machine to something that is polite, concise, enticing, and something that really markets your services. Set up your fax machine to do broadcasting, create a professional looking fax advertising your business, and send it out.

My Goals

____

____

____

What's in my way?

____

____

____

What action can I take to remedy the situation?

____

____

____

One-Year Progress Update Date ______________

____

____

____

POSITIVE AFFIRMATION: **I use my telephone as a marketing tool in the best possible ways.**

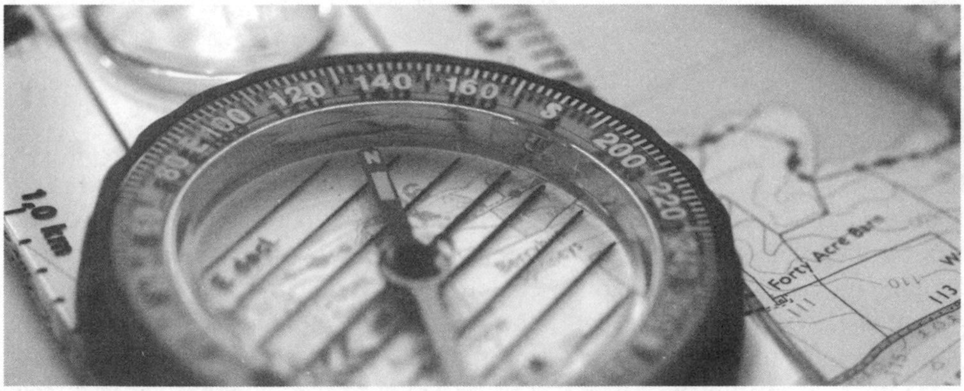

CHAPTER

10

Taking Care of Yourself

Never continue in a job you don't enjoy. If you're happy in what you're doing, you'll like yourself, you'll have inner peace. And if you have that, along with physical health, you will have had more success than you can possibly imagine.

—Johnny Carson

How is taking care of yourself important to building a successful massage practice? Because if you don't, you can't function at optimal performance, maintaining the vital balance of body, mind, and spirit.

We tell our clients to drink more water, to stretch, to exercise, to get regular massage. Are *you* doing that? The very nature of what we do is taking care of people. You can't take care of anyone unless you take care of yourself first.

Heather's Story

I trade massage with a couple of different therapists and never go more than two weeks without one. I also take a belly dancing class and a T'ai Chi class every week. I normally do 25–30 massages every week, and I realized early on that if I am going to keep up the pace I have set for myself in order to meet my financial goals, I have to make time for myself, and I don't let anything interfere with that.

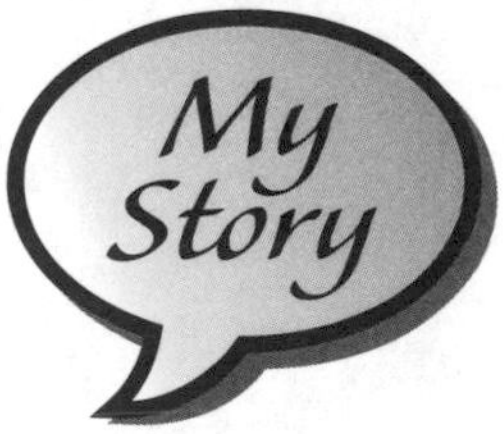

Building a successful business requires commitment, time, money, and most importantly, effort. Following the strategies in this book is going to require energy, hard work, and self-discipline. If you are in top form, it'll all be easier. When you come to work every day, with your eye on the prize of building the business you want, let your intent be to increase your prosperity and to have fun while going it. You can't do that if you're physically run down and mentally stressed out.

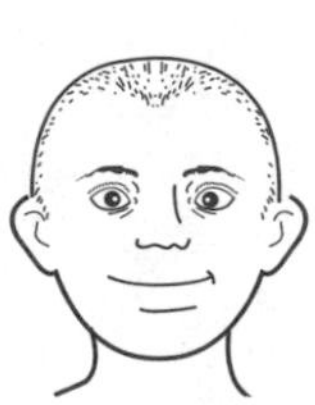

If it's been more than a month since you had a massage, call a fellow therapist right now and arrange a trade, or go pay for one. Do whatever you have to do. How can you look a client in the eye and tell them they need a massage every week if you're going a year without? That's pretty cheeky, and it verges on being unethical, too.

Any business owner will tell you that being self-employed is 24/7, and it is, but somewhere during that 24/7, there has to be time for you. You may have a spouse and/or children at home, be taking classes, be like a lot of therapists and still working at another job while you try to slowly build your practice, have housekeeping chores, grocery shopping, church and school activities, and some days you're just doing the best you can. When you're trying to build a business, you're worrying about money, bills, and manifesting enough prosperity.

Set a time every week, even if it's just an hour (just enough time for a massage) that is *your* time. Do something that refreshes and renews you, whether it's a nap or a trip to the beauty salon or an hour of reading that novel you've been putting off. Don't work seven days a week. If you can't make a living in six, you're not going to do it in seven, either. That's not meant to discourage you from working hard, but you have to play, too. A sharp mind is one that gets enough rest. You want your work to feed your spirit and your body to feel pleasantly tired at the end of the day, as if it is acknowledging that you did a good day's work—but not collapsing from exhaustion. Pace yourself.

If you're a new practitioner, and young to boot, you might think it's cool to massage 12 people in a day and make a big pile of money. Believe me, that won't last long. Your career is over if you blow out your thumbs from thinking you have to go to the bone on every client. Enthusiasm is a beautiful thing, but don't let it override your common sense. Leave enough time between appointments so you can change the table, deal with payment and rescheduling, and have enough time to pause, breathe, and refresh yourself without having to rush. Make a space in your daily schedule for a healthy sit-down lunch instead of gulping a few swallows of junk food between appointments. A stressed out therapist is hardly in a position to help a stressed out client!

Taking care of yourself also means practicing good body mechanics and having your workspace set up with the intent that it is ergonomically efficient. Having your table set at the correct height, having things arranged so that what you use regularly is within easy reach, and removing any potential hazards will make your workday less tiring.

Finally, and this is just my theory—not a scientific fact—have fun at work! Taking care of yourself means watching out for your physical health and safety, of course, but your mental health is every bit as important, if not more so. Laugh out loud every day. Dr. Harry Walker, a favorite former teacher and mentor of mine, used to open his classes with having everyone stand up and belly laugh. For the first couple of seconds, people felt awkward about laughing for no reason other than the joy of laughing, but within thirty seconds, you couldn't stop if you wanted to. It is a very wonderful stress reliever. Read something spiritual and uplifting every day, even if it's just a one-liner. Listen to uplifting music. Repeat positive affirmations, or meditate, or both. Feed your soul with something that's important to you. It has already been suggested that you perform a marketing activity every day. Do something to take care of yourself every day, too.

My Personal Journey

This Week's Activity: Taking Care of Myself

Date ____________________

For this week's activity, set some goals for taking care of yourself. Make a standing appointment to trade massage with another practitioner. Set aside some personal downtime to unwind from the pressures of studying, school, business, and whatever else consumes most of your time. Find an activity that relaxes and restores you and devote some time to that on a regular basis.

My Goals

____

____

____

What's in my way?

____

____

____

What action can I take to remedy the situation?

____

____

____

One-Year Progress Update

Date ____________________

____

____

____

POSITIVE AFFIRMATION: **Taking care of myself enables me to care for others.**

PART 3

The Path to Promotion

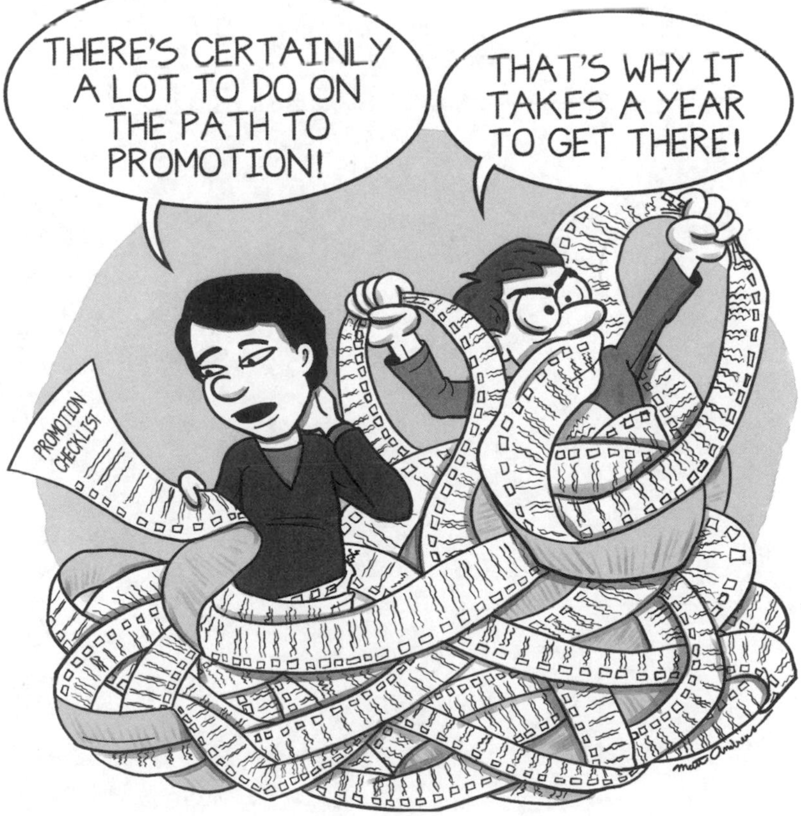

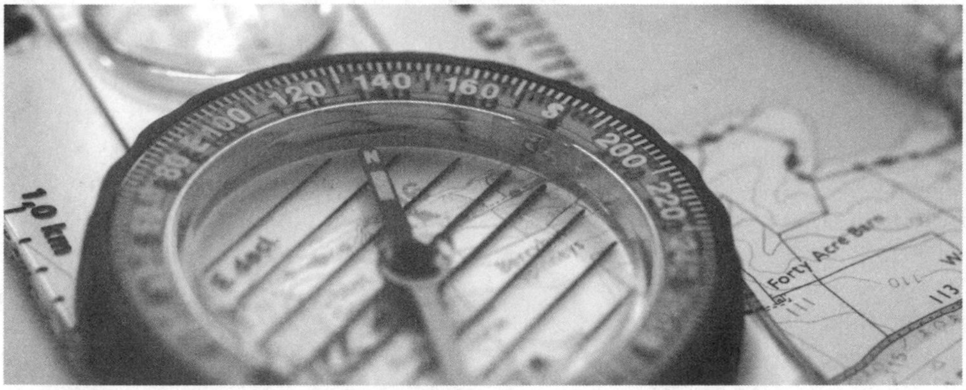

CHAPTER 11

Join a Professional Association

A man is a success if he gets up in the morning, goes to bed at night and in between does what he wants to do.

—Bob Dylan

There are several national and international associations for massage therapists. In addition to providing liability insurance for practitioners, these associations each have various benefits to the membership. The major organizations in the United States are the American Massage Therapy Association (AMTA) and Associated Bodywork and Massage Professionals (ABMP). There is also the American Massage Council.

In addition to these, there are associations that are for practitioners of specific disciplines, such as the International Reiki Practitioner Association, the Reflexology Association of America, the American Polarity Association, and others specific in nature. There are also other organizations that are broader in scope that massage therapists are welcome to join, such as the American Holistic Health Association, the American Association of Drugless Practitioners, and others.

Membership in the National Certification Board for Therapeutic Massage & Bodywork (NCBTMB) is limited to those practitioners who have passed the National Certification Exam (NCE) in Massage Therapy, or Massage Therapy and Bodywork. As of press time, 32 states and the District of Columbia use the NCE as their measure of competence in order to qualify for licensure. In the states that have no licensure, many practitioners still choose to become nationally certified in order to advance their identity as a professional massage therapist and to set themselves apart from those who have no training, but call themselves massage therapists—an all too common problem in states with no requirements. A therapist must have at least 500 hours of education that includes theory and practice of massage and bodywork, anatomy, physiology, kinesiology, pathology, business practices, and professional ethics before being allowed to sit for the exam. The NCBTMB is not in the insurance business.

One of the benefits to membership these organizations have in common are practitioner locator or referral services on the Internet, allowing the public to search for therapists by state, city, specialty, and so forth. Many also provide a toll-free number for clients searching for massage therapists, and therapists seeking support. This benefit alone can generate enough business to offset the cost of your membership.

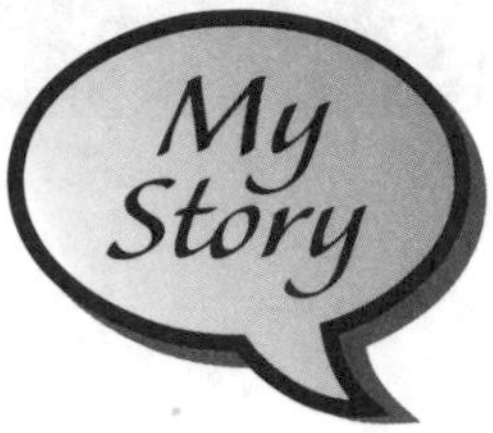

Lynne's Story

I joined a professional association as soon as I became a student and have been an active member ever since. I have attended a lot of Continuing Ed workshops and conventions, served as a volunteer in several capacities, and met a lot of great people. I had the chance to do massage at the Olympics, and my local chapter raised money to fund my trip, an opportunity I otherwise would not have had. I definitely feel belonging is worth my annual dues for the benefits I receive.

Some of the organizations are providers of continuing education approved by state and/or national boards. Members are offered the opportunity to attend low-cost classes that are subsidized by their membership fees. Other benefits include such varied things as journal and newsletter subscriptions, the right to use the organization's logo on your business literature, access to research databases, free or reasonably priced websites and/or links, free classified ads and job bulletin boards, chat rooms for practitioners, discounts on massage equipment and supplies, and more. AMTA, for instance, is a non-profit entity that supports research in addition to subsidizing education. In the aftermath of the devastation of Hurricanes Katrina and Rita in the Gulf states in 2005, AMTA assisted several hundred massage therapists who had lost everything with practice rebuilding kits and dues relief.

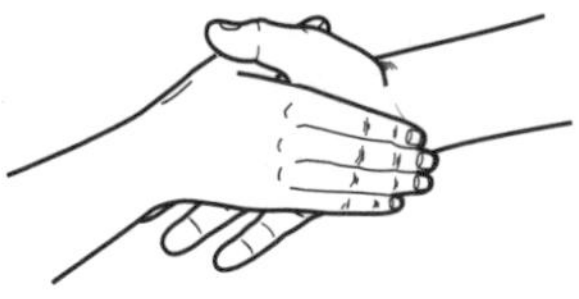

Two of the associations that I belong to have biannual statewide and annual nationwide conventions, and one of the international associations also has an annual convention. These are huge networking opportunities. I live in North Carolina, but as a result of meeting people at conventions, I have had people from as far away as Iowa, California, and Canada attend my continuing education classes. I have also met therapists from Los Angeles, Boca Raton, Albuquerque, and Washington, D.C. that I was able to refer my clients to when they moved to those cities, and dozens I can refer to in other areas of my own state. I've met therapists from other places that I have been able to get a short notice appointment with when I was passing through their state. I've formed friendships with therapists from the other side of the world, gotten jobs teaching massage in other states and in Europe, and been able to bring other teachers in from other states and countries to teach at my facility through networking.

Don't overlook the fact that travel to and from, and any costs associated with attending conventions, continuing education classes, and professional meetings are tax deductible. It's a sweet thing to take a class on a cruise ship or at a nice resort from a top-notch massage instructor and write it off on your income tax. Many times these opportunities cost less than you think. Several of the more well known teachers and authors in our profession regularly teach on cruises or other trips at very reasonable prices.

Some associations also have volunteer opportunities that can advance your career. Volunteering at the local, state, or national level of your association is not only a satisfying way to be in service and to learn something new, it can also be worth a press release or media appearance that will show you and your business in a positive, professional light. Hopefully, nobody volunteers just so they can see their name in the paper—but when it happens, savor the moment. Volunteering is a good way to give back to the profession, and again, an invaluable networking opportunity.

Don't be guilty of just paying your insurance money to the professional association and not doing anything else—don't let your membership be a wasted opportunity! Participate in all the activities that you can and attend all the meetings that you can. Write an article for the organization's magazine or newsletter, and if you can't write, at least read what other people have contributed. Take advantage of the research databases to keep up on the latest developments in massage and bodywork. Attend the classes they offer—or teach one, if you have something to offer. Network, network, and network some more. Make it a point to learn something from every contact you make, and be willing to share your own experiences with others. You'll get your membership investment back many times over.

My Personal Journey

This Week's Activity: Joining a Professional Association Date ____________________

For this week's activity, make it a point to join at least one professional association—and be a proactive member. If you are already a member of one of the professional associations, review the benefits you are entitled to as a member, such as free internet listings, continuing education opportunities, newsletters, volunteer participation, and so forth, to be sure that you are maximizing the benefits of your membership in order to help your business grow.

My Goals

____

____

____

What's in my way?

____

____

____

What action can I take to remedy the situation?

____

____

____

One-Year Progress Update Date ____________________

____

____

____

POSITIVE AFFIRMATION: **I take advantage of my professional associations in order to help my practice grow to its fullest potential.**

CHAPTER

12

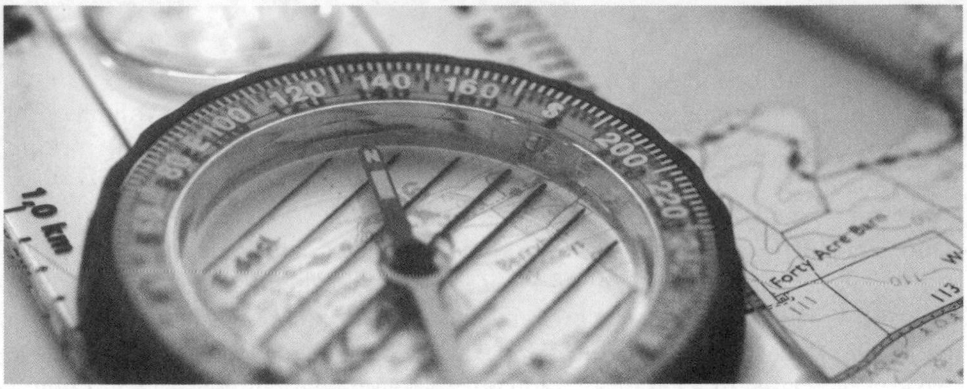

Join the Chamber of Commerce

The only place success comes before work is the dictionary.

—Vidal Sassoon

Membership in the Chamber of Commerce in your community is one of the best investments in terms of value and return that you can make. I feel that I must share the credit for the success of my business with our local Chamber.

As soon as I opened my business, a representative of the Chamber came to visit and asked me to join. For $130 per year, this is what I got:

The chamber organized a ribbon-cutting ceremony for my business. They took care of inviting local dignitaries, like the mayor, the town council, the chief of police, and the president of a local radio station. The local newspaper came and took a picture of the event at no cost. Besides appearing in the newspaper, the picture was also inserted into a publication the Chamber puts out four times a year about our county, and these are distributed at the Chamber itself, the two welcome centers in the county (our county borders the state line), and other various venues, again at no cost.

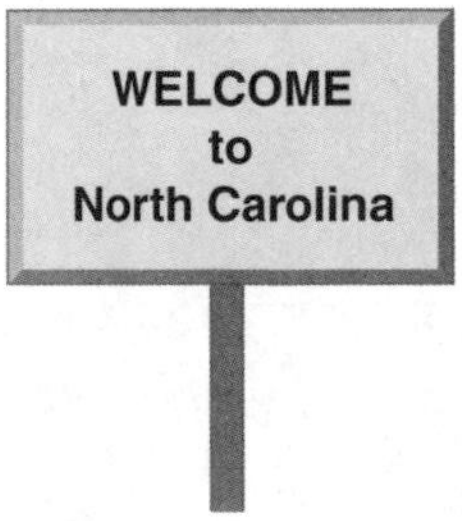

Upon joining, I was also given discounts for 50% off on advertising with the local newspaper, a local free shopper paper with a circulation of about 10,000, the local cable television company, and the local radio station. I didn't waste those on small ads. For 50% off, I splurged and got big ones that I otherwise couldn't have afforded when I was just starting out.

The Chamber also promotes a "meet and greet" each month, called "Business After Hours," held at different businesses, and the turnouts are great. People come to check out your business and what you have to offer, have a snack and a drink, and network. The Chamber executives attend, and they do everything they can to publicize these events.

The first time I hosted "Business After Hours," the turnout was miraculous; more than fifty people piled into our office. I was so impressed with the number of people who came by to see my business that I wrote a letter of thanks to the Chamber president, thanking them for supporting my business and publicizing this great way to introduce myself to the community. The result of that was, the president called me and wanted my permission to copy my letter in an advertisement to run in the newspaper. It was a big ad on the second page of the newspaper, and there was my letter prominently displayed in the middle of it, again at no cost.

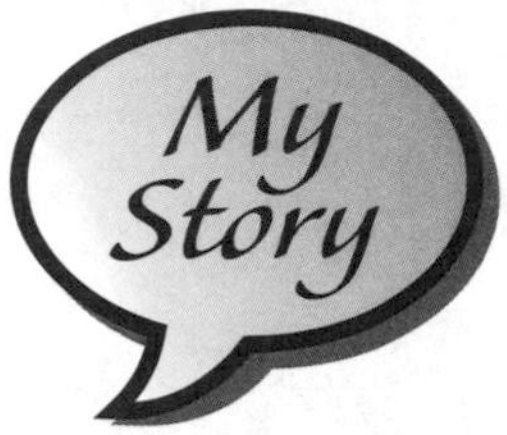

Todd's Story

I had been in business for about a year and was really struggling to make ends meet. Ironically, my office was just around the corner from the Chamber of Commerce, but I didn't join because I convinced myself I needed to spend the money elsewhere. My cousin, a Chamber member, finally convinced me that I had to join and be an active member. My business picked up instantly! I started going to Chamber events and meeting other business people and attending the workshops they hold for small business people. If I had it to do over, I'd have joined my first day in business.

Not only did my own "Business After Hours" produce a great turnout, I make it a point to attend as many as I can that other businesses host. These events are simply great opportunities to meet other business people in the community and promote your business.

Another therapist I am acquainted with owns a very successful spa in a large city. She can afford to pay for all the advertising she wants, but she couldn't have done any better than this—she wrote a letter thanking her local Chamber for support, and they asked her permission to print it in the *national* Chamber of Commerce newspaper. As a result of *that* appearance, she was contacted by a luxury travel magazine, which featured her spa in an article about her city. She got free publicity all over the country just for writing a simple thank-you letter.

The Chamber constantly sponsors seminars to educate and inform small business people. One of this year's events was called "The Panel of Experts," and it took place at the local community college. Topics on many subjects of concern to small business people were covered, including applying for loans, tax strategies, and so forth, and they asked me to conduct a seminar on stress management. The result of that was that my picture and the name of my business appeared on the front page of the newspaper before the event, along with the other presenters, and a nice paragraph about my teaching massage and other techniques for stress management, again at no cost. After the event, there was another article in the paper about what a success the event was, and my name and the business name were mentioned again, at no cost.

The Chamber sends out e-mail and fax notices once or twice a week to inform the membership of these seminars, meet and greets, and anything else of interest that is happening. The Chamber hosts numerous events throughout the year as fundraisers, including a golf tournament, an annual barbeque, street festivals in the spring and the fall, and a reverse raffle at Christmas that is a fancy-dress affair. Participating in these events means more networking opportunities and more free publicity. Donate a massage and you'll be listed as a sponsor or donor in ads and printed programs. During the street festivals, we always set up a booth on the courthouse lawn and do free chair massage, and it is the most popular booth at the festival. It's

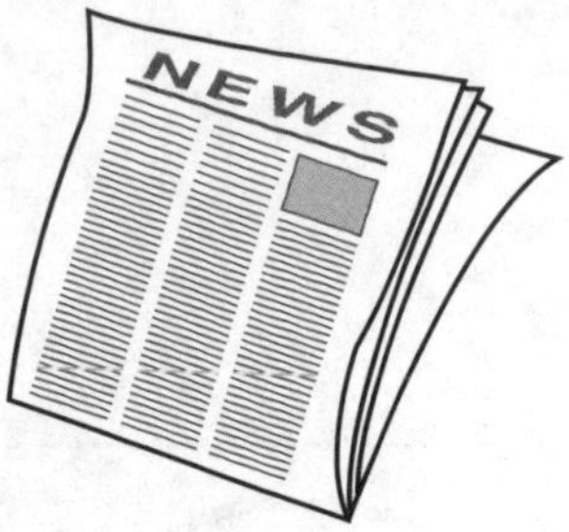

almost guaranteed that we're going to get our picture in the paper, again at no cost, and even if we don't, we've still introduced our business to hundreds of potential new customers.

Another benefit to Chamber membership is low-cost access to their mailing list of all members. Address labels for our local 500+ membership is $20. Fax-on-demand is even less. You can let other businesses know about your event or specials very cheaply. The Chamber also has a program called member-to-member, which encourages member businesses to give discounts to each other.

Our local Chamber has a very impressive website that businesses are listed on at no extra charge as a member benefit, and it links with our own website. The Chamber office itself, which is on Main Street, has a huge display area for any member business to place business cards, brochures, and so forth, and they also solicit literature that they personally deliver to the state welcome centers and the tourism development office.

In summary, it's hard to imagine anything that can help your business more for the least amount of money than joining the Chamber of Commerce. I have talked to therapists in other towns and cities who assure me that my experience is not unique, and that the chambers in their towns also provide many marketing opportunities that are low-cost and no-cost in exchange for their nominal membership fee. If your town does not have a Chamber of Commerce, there is usually a Merchant's Association that is a similar organization. They are there to support businesses, and they do a great job. Join, and be an active member. You'll be glad you did.

My Personal Journey

This Week's Activity: Joining the Chamber of Commerce Date ____________

For this week's activity, you are going to investigate the benefits of joining the Chamber of Commerce in your town. If you are already a professional therapist and you don't yet belong, give serious consideration to joining. If you are a student, you can still visit the Chamber and find out about the benefits of becoming a member once you are a professional. Make a list of the pros and cons—cost vs. benefits of membership—and what you stand to lose if you don't join. If you are already a member and you have not been an active participant in Chamber activities, resolve to change that now and become proactive in your membership.

My Goals

____

____

____

What's in my way?

____

____

____

What action can I take to remedy the situation?

____

____

____

One-Year Progress Update Date ____________

____

____

____

POSITIVE AFFIRMATION: **I actively participate in organizations that can help my business grow.**

CHAPTER

13

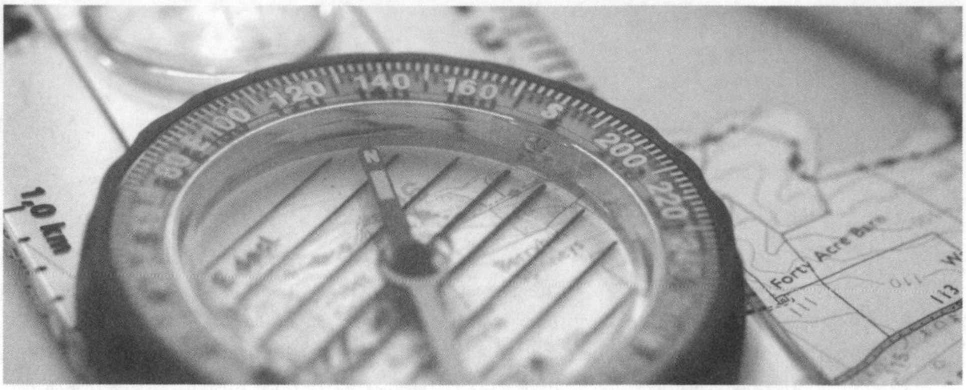

Payment Options for Your Clients

What is success? I think it is a mixture of having a flair for the thing that you are doing; knowing that it is not enough, that you have got to have hard work and a certain sense of purpose.

—MARGARET THATCHER

Providing several payment options for your clients is a marketing strategy that works. If you're only accepting cash, it's time to rethink that decision. The American public has grown to expect that credit and debit cards will be accepted everywhere. Accepting personal checks is a courtesy to the client and a risk to you. So are other options, like offering payment plans and accepting insurance clients. There is a certain amount of risk, and in the case of credit cards, a certain amount of expense that will be incurred if you decide to conduct business this way. On the other hand, offering your clients a variety of ways to pay virtually insures that you will have a lot more business than you would as a strictly cash operator.

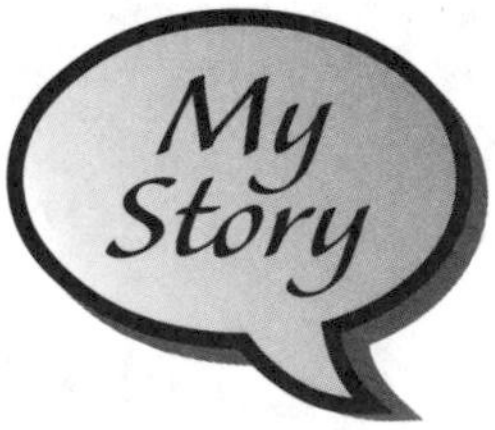

Nadia's Story

When I started accepting credit cards, it was near the end of my second year in business. It has been very easy for me to see that the sales of gift certificates and packages have increased greatly since I started accepting the cards.

Credit Cards

The fact is that America is a credit-card society. Although some people would charge the massage because they don't have the cash on hand at the moment, others would charge just because they charge everything they can to build up frequent

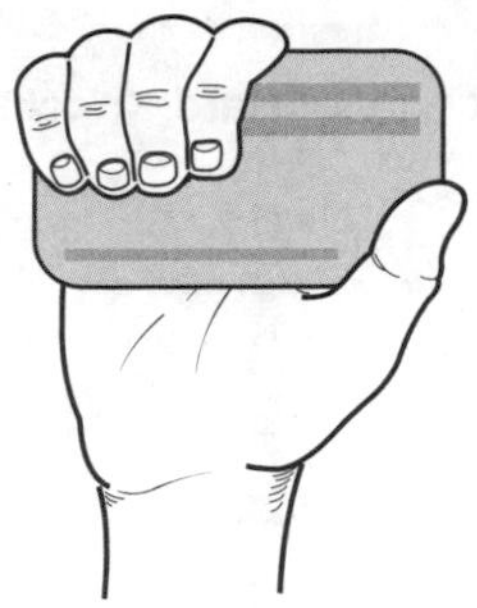

flyer miles or other rewards. One therapist I know says she refuses to take credit cards because she doesn't want to contribute to people's debt. That is not her decision to make, and she is taking the decision away from the consumer.

Accepting credit cards (and announcing that option) can bring an immediate increase in clients. There is a downside; it costs *you* money to accept cards. Each credit card issuer sets their own percentage rate that they will charge you for processing their cards. In addition to that, there may also be a per-item charge. In an average month, my business incurs about $150 in credit card fees. During the Christmas season, that can go as high as $500 because of our package and gift certificate sales. Additionally, when I first started the business, I did not have the cash to purchase the credit-card machine, which at that time was around $1,200. Instead, I signed a 36-month lease that costs me $37 per month. Sure enough, that cost me about $133 more to handle it that way. On the upside, if it breaks, the company will replace it for free. And, when the 36 months is up, they'll offer to sell it to me at a reduced price, or give me a discount to purchase or lease a new one, because they'd like to keep me as a customer after all the money I've sent their way. In just a short few years, the credit business has changed to the point that most credit-card processors will no longer charge you for the machine. They'll actually give it to you to keep as long as you do business with them.

Personal Checks

Taking personal checks seems risky to some therapists. They are worried about bouncing checks and being short on money. Although there will always be one or two unscrupulous people who write bad checks, it is really a relatively rare occurrence, at least at my business. Most banks now have a toll-free check verification number you can call to make sure the check is good. Some credit card machines even allow you to scan checks on the spot, or you can ask for a debit card instead of a paper check. A lot of the merchants in my area now have a sign posted at the cash register informing patrons that their check is going to be scanned and that the money will be deducted from their account at that very moment. That deters people who might be tempted to write a bad check with the intent of getting their money to the bank before it clears.

Consider the circumstances. If the client is a regular customer, you should certainly have enough confidence in them to take their check. If she is someone new that you hope to gain as a regular customer, refusing her check is not going to endear you to her. If she's a tourist from out of town that you never expect to see again, you are definitely within your rights to politely explain that you don't accept out-of-town checks. Anecdotally, in the past three years I have only had two bad checks. One of them was from another massage therapist who had a mistake in her checkbook; the other was from someone who worked in another office in our building—not two people that I would have pegged as likely to write a bad check. The therapist made good on it. The company the other person worked for moved out of the building to the next town and I decided it wasn't worth my time to go to court and expend my energy over $50.

If you decide to accept personal checks, you need to have a policy posted. It may be in the form of a sign on the wall or a statement on your printed receipts, that checks returned for insufficient funds will be subject to additional fees, and cost of court should that become necessary. I decided not to blow a day in court over $50, but if that customer had written a bad check for $400 to pay for a full day of spa treatments, I wouldn't have let that slide. Your bank probably charges you a fee for processing a bad check through your account and you have to recoup that from the client—assuming you can get them to pay it. Anyone can make an honest mistake, and I like to give people the benefit of the doubt before I threaten

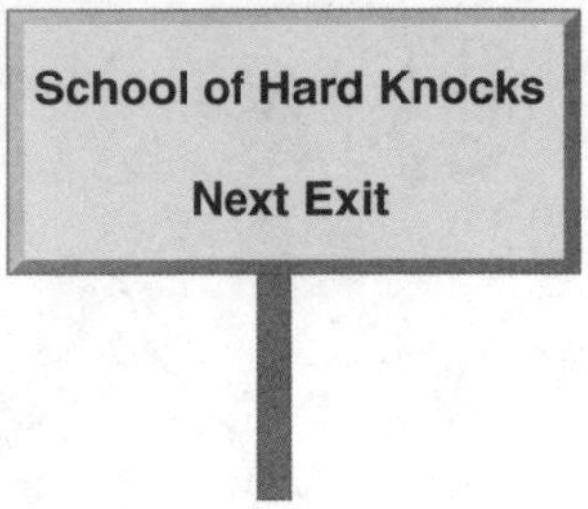

them with legal action. I later found out that the person who had written the $50 check had done the same thing to other merchants all over town. She knew when she wrote the check that it was not good and in fact the account was closed. I didn't call the merchant line to verify the check when she gave it to me because I knew her parents very well, and it just never occurred to me that their daughter was a crook—a nice lesson for me.

Payment Plans

Along with the convenience of being able to pay by credit card and personal check, you may consider having payment plans. Payment plans are something you should not do unless you can afford to wait a little while for your money, but if you feel inclined to help someone, a payment plan can be a blessing for them. Say you've seen a new client who really needs a lot of bodywork, but they can only afford to come twice a month. You just don't feel that they're going to get better going that route, so you could offer them a payment plan—financing their treatment for them, charging a little interest for the convenience to them, if they will agree to come every week for eight weeks, or whatever you think they need. You will want to avoid payment plans until you're more well established and your bank account won't feel the squeeze, or at least be cautious about how many you take at one time. Extending this courtesy to people generates good will and they'll remember that you helped them in their time of need.

If you do decide to offer anyone a payment plan, get it in writing. Here is a sample:

Installment Payment Agreement

I, ________________, agree that I will pay Laura Allen, Licensed Massage Therapist, in the amount of $75 per month for my treatment until such time as all treatments I have received are paid for. I understand that I am scheduled for four sessions of massage therapy per month for two months at a cost of $60 per session, bringing my total indebtedness to $480, plus 5% interest on the unpaid balance, compounded monthly. I understand that this is a binding contract and that my failure to pay this debt by the terms agreed upon will result in legal action being taken against me.

Signed ________________________________ Date ____________________

Laura Allen, LMBT ________________________ Date ____________________

Accepting Insurance

Many insurance companies still haven't caught on to the fact that if they'd pay for massage, they'd save millions on pills and surgery. Some, however, have decided it's time to wake up and smell the coffee. Advertising the fact that you accept insurance can mean an instant influx of clients.

One caveat—you have to be in a cash flow position to wait for the majority of your money. Most insurance plans require a co-payment. On a $50 or $60 massage you might receive $10-20 from the client at the time of service, and you'll be waiting for the rest. Please don't do this until you can afford it. There have been times when I was waiting to be paid for 70 claims. In fact, at this very moment, I am owed around $8,000 by insurance companies. I have already paid my staff members to do those massages, and I am the one waiting for the money. If you're not financially prepared to have that kind of money on the accounts receivable side of your balance sheet, don't start taking insurance until you are. Once you're entrenched in the system, the money from the insurance companies flows in fairly regularly, but when you first sign on you may expect a couple of months waiting to be paid. If you can't afford to wait, you can always offer clients the option that they pay you up front and have the insurance company reimburse them.

Accepting insurance also means paperwork. Be sure you have the time and expertise to fill out the necessary Health Insurance Claim Form (HICF), which is a standardized thing in the U.S. Insurance companies also have the expectation that you are keeping professional SOAP notes and that you will provide them with progress notes for every patient. They expect that every i will be dotted and every t will be crossed, that you are using correct procedure and diagnosis codes (which you will obtain from the referring physician—*you* are not diagnosing anyone), and so forth. Remember, too, that insurance companies are in the business of avoiding paying as many claims as possible. It's a double-edged sword.

Never perform work on an insurance client without calling their insurance company for authorization—most of the time, they will tell you immediately before giving you the authorization code that a phone authorization is no guarantee of payment. Many times, a doctor's prescription will be required before an insurance company will pay. Some companies require an authorization for every single visit, while others will tell you on the first call that they are authorizing *x* number of visits during a certain time frame.

As above for the payment plan, you will want to have the client sign a practitioner's lien, stating that in the event the insurance company doesn't pay, that they acknowledge that they are responsible and agree to pay the full amount. Here is an example:

Practitioner's Lien

Main Street Massage, 250 Main Street, Cliffden, North Carolina, 28199

I, ______________, hereby acknowledge that Main Street Massage is filing (an) insurance claim(s) on my behalf. I understand that a representative of Main Street Massage has contacted my insurance company for prior authorization to perform treatment procedures, with the understanding that prior authorization is not a guarantee of payment. I agree that in the event said insurance company fails to pay Main Street Massage within 90 days for any reason that I am liable in full for any and all monies owed to Main Street Massage. I understand that should it become necessary, Main Street Massage will use all legal means at their disposal to collect such monies, and that any costs of legal representation and costs of court will also be my responsibility. I understand that the therapists at Main Street Massage are performing services for me in good faith and that they have the legal right to expect payment for their services. I understand that I am at risk of having a lien placed on my personal property and/or garnishment of wages if I fail to meet my financial obligation to Main Street Massage.

Signature______________________________ Date ____________________

Representative of Main Street Massage Signature____________________

Insurance companies are also sticklers for having a W-9 form from the practitioner, which gives them either your social security number, or your employer identification number, depending upon how your business is set up. It doesn't matter if that number is on every other piece of paper you send them; they still want the form. If you want to get into the insurance game, it would be prudent on your part to go take a class in billing insurance. If you can't find a nearby class, there are home study courses available, or you could call your doctor or chiropractor's office and offer one of the billing clerks a free massage or two, to show you how to do things properly so you'll get paid.

If you have the fortitude to deal with the paperwork, and the money to sustain yourself while getting into the insurance loop, you can get to the point of having to put potential clients on a waiting list much faster than you'd expect. When I first started accepting insurance, I quickly had a domino effect—the first customer from a manufacturing facility that had an insurance plan covering massage must have gone back to the factory and told everyone there they needed a massage and that the insurance company was going to pay for it. Within two weeks, we got thirty new clients, and the same can easily happen for you. Just be sure you can stay afloat while you wait for the claims to be paid.

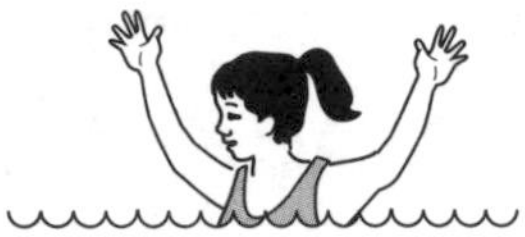

There are two other caveats about insurance: Workers' Compensation and personal injury claims. The laws governing Workers' Compensation may vary from state to state. In our state, it is against the law for a therapist to bill the client for whatever portion of the bill the Workers' Compensation does not cover. The clincher is that they won't tell you up front how much they're going to pay. You basically agree that you will accept whatever that amount is. I have done $1,000 worth of work on a Workers' Compensation case and only received $350 for it. I was not happy. I no longer accept those cases, and I will not accept a personal injury case on a contingency basis anymore, either. In a personal injury case, you agree that you will wait for a lawsuit to be settled to collect your money. I have two cases on my books worth several thousand dollars right now that are more than five years old and they still aren't settled. There have been many times when I could have used that money.

To summarize, the more ways you have available for people to pay you, the more business you can cultivate. Sometimes a payment option is the difference in whether a potential customer chooses to patronize your business, or someone else's.

Your Cancellation Policy

While we are discussing payment options for your clients, we should also touch on what you are going to do to about cancelled appointments. If you are just starting out as a sole proprietor, maybe you haven't yet considered the need to have a cancellation policy. You may be the type to give everyone the benefit of a doubt—that if someone didn't show up and didn't call, it must have been an emergency; otherwise, they wouldn't blow you off without calling. Let me impart some wisdom from my years of experience: people do it all the time, and they don't give it a second thought. Of course, your regular clients are not usually going to be the ones to do this to you—but even a regular isn't above having a forgetful moment. It's a wise idea to give people an appointment card and a reminder call the day before the appointment. The dilemma here is to charge or not to charge for cancelled appointments.

It's a wise idea to have a written cancellation policy right on your intake form and to ask the client to initial it, proving that they have been informed of your policy. In my office, everyone is allowed one no-show per year without being penalized. More than one and they're going to be billed for the appointment. If they don't pay, they aren't welcome to come back unless they guarantee the visit with a credit card. If you're fortunate enough to be a busy therapist, you may even have people on a waiting list hoping someone cancels so they can get in with you. If a client does a no-show, you don't have any opportunity to give that appointment away to someone who wishes they could have it. And yes of course, I realize that everyone has the occasional crisis, such as a death in the family, which might cause them to forget an appointment. I do make allowances for such circumstances.

Some therapists (and most doctors' offices) request a 24-hour notice of cancellation. At my office, we request four hours. That gives us enough time to call someone on the waiting list and give them the opportunity to take the appointment. If someone has abused your good nature one too many times in the past, consider asking them to guarantee their appointment with a credit card. You can set your own policy. And don't forget, it's always within your discretion to turn down appointments with such people. You don't have to accuse them of anything; all you have to do is say, "I'm sorry, I'm totally booked right now."

If you are employed by someone, you probably have no say-so over the payment methods available or the cancellation policy. It's a wise move, when seeking employment, to clarify what the cancellation policy is and whether or not you can expect any compensation for missed appointments.

Offering your clients a number of different payment options is a service to them. Protecting your income by having a cancellation policy is a service you need to perform for yourself. A therapist I know who works in a physician's office told me recently that the doctor bills patients for the missed appointments—but doesn't pass that money on to her. It's a good idea to have the terms of your employment and such circumstances clarified in writing.

My Personal Journey

This Week's Activity: To Expand My Payment Options Date ____________________

For this week's activity, work on expanding the payment options available to your clients. Call a minimum of three credit card processing companies; let them know that you are actively seeking the best deal available for your business and that you will be calling their competitors. Consider taking a class in filing insurance claims, or ask another practitioner who's already accepting insurance to help you get started. Let your clients know through e-mail, direct mail, and a sign in your office that you now have several payment options available. Also write your cancellation policy.

My Goals

____

____

____

What's in my way?

____

____

____

What action can I take to remedy the situation?

____

____

____

One-Year Progress Update Date ____________________

____

____

____

POSITIVE AFFIRMATION: **Offering options to my clients brings me personal prosperity.**

CHAPTER 14

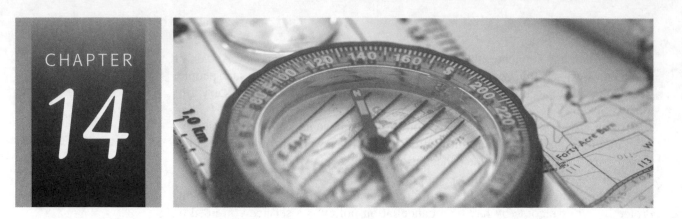

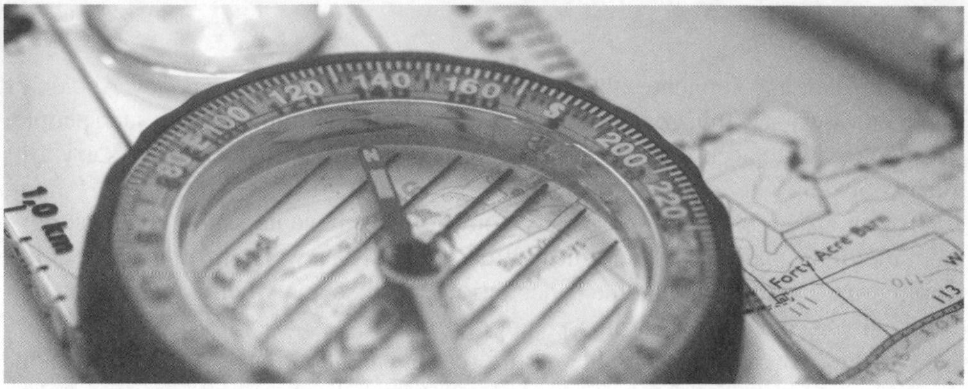

Your Mailing List

Nothing succeeds like the appearance of success.

—Christopher Lasch

Developing Your Own List

You've got your client database or files, so that's your mailing list, right? Wrong! That's a *part* of your mailing list. The objective of this book is to get you new clients. While we certainly want to keep the old ones happy, mailing *only* to them will probably not bring in that much new business.

Any time you are at a community service event, have a sign-in sheet. Ask for name, address, phone, and e-mail. Include a disclaimer that you will not share their information with anyone, and when asking for e-mail, state "if you would like to be notified by e-mail of specials and events" so people will not think you're spamming them.

Working a street festival? Put out a bucket or fishbowl and entry tickets for someone to win a free massage. Same deal—on the tickets get their name, address, phone, and e-mail.

My Story

Kim Lee's Story

I carry a small notebook in my purse all the time for collecting names and addresses. Not only do I add to my mailing list in the usual ways of collecting names at community service events and the like, I try to add anyone new that I meet anywhere! I view every new contact as a potential client or referral source. When I am talking to them about my business, I just ask them if they would like to be added to my mailing list. Most people say yes, and I use that opportunity to send them a discount coupon for their first massage. I get lots of new people that way.

Collect names for your mailing list any time you are at any event away from your office. Don't forget about in the office—lots of times people who are not yet customers themselves come in to buy a gift certificate for someone or just to ask questions about your services. While they're here, ask them if they'd like to be put on your mailing list for your free newsletter. Keeping a clipboard right on your desk is great for this purpose—just put a note at the top that existing clients will automatically be placed on the list and don't have to sign up. It's also handy if you carry a little notebook or one of those handheld personal computers. Let's say you've met someone and given them your elevator speech—you can always end that by asking if they'd like to be added to your mailing list.

The mailing list made up of non-clients is going to be an ephemeral mailing list—it will need to be purged from time to time, and more added to it. For example, when I work a street festival or community service event and collect names, first I will send those people a discount postcard. Remember, I have collected their contact information by holding a drawing for a free massage. So I just make a postcard that says, "Thanks for stopping at the THERA-SSAGE booth at the Octoberfest. Bring this card in for $10 off on your first massage."

I also send them a copy of our latest newsletter (by e-mail, if they provided that address). That's two pieces of mail. If I haven't had any response by the time the next newsletter comes out, I purge them from the list. Of course they may still come in some time in the future, but I'm not going to spend any more time or money soliciting them. Two contacts is enough. I also maintain the currency of my list by having "Address Service Requested" printed on all materials that I mail to clients. That means the post office will provide me with their new address, even if the forwarding order has expired, and that I will receive the card back notifying me in the event the person has moved and left no forwarding address. The charge per piece is very minimal and keeps me from wasting postage by mailing people again who no longer have a valid address on file.

Lists From Other Sources

If you belong to the Chamber of Commerce or Merchant's Association in your town, you can probably purchase their mailing list at a very cheap cost. There are also plenty of companies that sell mailing lists of general and specific interest, broken down by zip codes, and so forth. For instance, you can purchase a list of people who have shown previous interest in holistic health in your area. These tend to be expensive and are probably best avoided, unless you have a lot of discretionary money.

Don't share your mailing list with anyone. First, it's a violation of confidentiality, which as massage therapists we are bound to. It's an invasion of people's privacy. The same with those computer programs that harvest the address of everyone who's visited your website. If those people had wanted you to contact them, they would have filled out your form—but they didn't—so don't spam them. You don't like it when it happens to you. If you teach Continuing Education, or if you retail products that would be of interest to other massage therapists, you can usually purchase the mailing lists of licensed therapists in your state from your state massage board. The National Certification Board for Therapeutic Massage and Bodywork also sells their mailing list, broken down by region, state, or zip code—or you can mail to every certified person in their database—if you have the money.

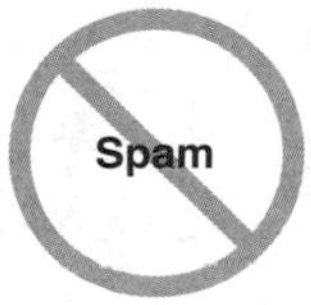

Direct Mailing

We've already mentioned mailing newsletters and coupons to customers or potential customers. Direct mailing should not be overlooked as a source of relatively cheap advertising. In addition to your newsletter, you can send out postcard notices

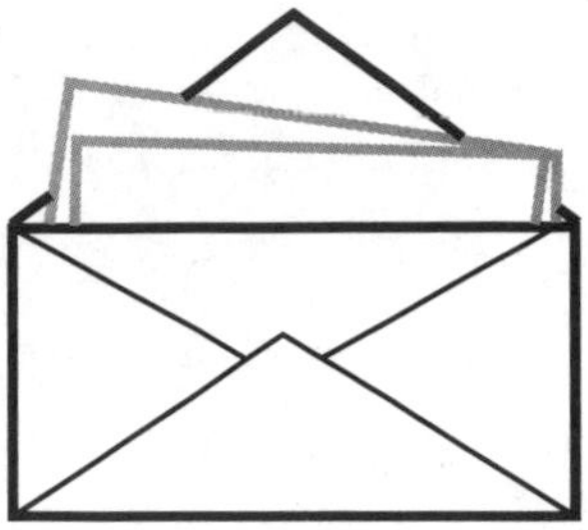

of specials you may be offering and health fairs or other events you will be hosting or appearing at. Let's talk about coupons for a minute. People often throw discount coupons in the trash—but they don't throw away gift certificates. If you do a mailing of that type, instead of having "$10 discount coupon" printed on it, call it a "$10 Gift Certificate." As a holiday that is typically a good gift certificate sales period draws near, try mailing out a page with three or four gift certificates on it—with instructions to call and receive an activation code for the certificates. These work best if they're attractive and in colored ink.

Depending on how long your client list is, it may serve you to do bulk mailings through the post office or another provider. Businesses such as Kinko's or Staples offer bulk mailing services for an additional fee if you don't mail regularly enough from the post office to warrant paying their annual charge for the service (the postage is extra). Your mailbox can and should be a great source of marketing opportunities for you.

My Personal Journey

This Week's Activity: Develop a Mailing List Date ____________

For this week's activity, start developing your mailing list, if you're still a student. If you are already practicing, review your mailing list and your procedures for maintaining it to make sure it is serving you as well as it can. Create a new and attractive sign-up list and use it from now on every time you attend a community service function, health fair, or other event where you could collect new addresses. Don't forget about your website; you can have people sign up for your mailing list right from your site.

My Goals

____

____

____

What's in my way?

____

____

____

What action can I take to remedy the situation?

____

____

____

One-Year Progress Update Date ____________

____

____

____

POSITIVE AFFIRMATION: **My mailing list keeps a river of clients flowing to me.**

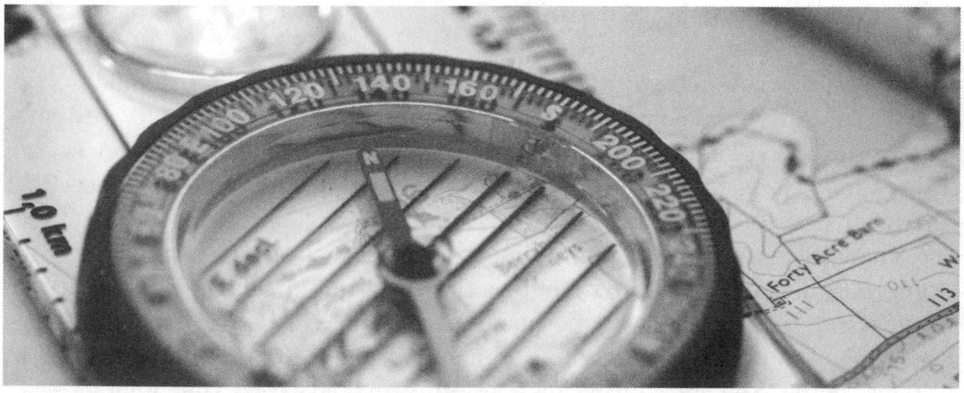

CHAPTER 15

A Grand Opening

The difference between a successful person and others is not a lack of strength, or a lack of knowledge, but rather in a lack of will.

—Vince Lombardi

If you are just opening your practice, plan to have a grand opening. If you have been in business for a while, just take the same concept and host an open house or a customer appreciation day.

For a first-time grand opening, your local newspaper will usually agree to come out and take a picture of your business or ribbon-cutting ceremony at no charge.

People love a party—but you have to get the word out. If you are new to the business and don't already have an established clientele, this is one of those occasions when you will have to spend some money to advertise the event. As I mentioned in Chapter 12, if you join the Chamber of Commerce, they will be glad to assist you with publicizing the event. Even so, you'll still want to advertise it in the newspaper, by direct mail, posting flyers on community bulletin boards, and any way you can.

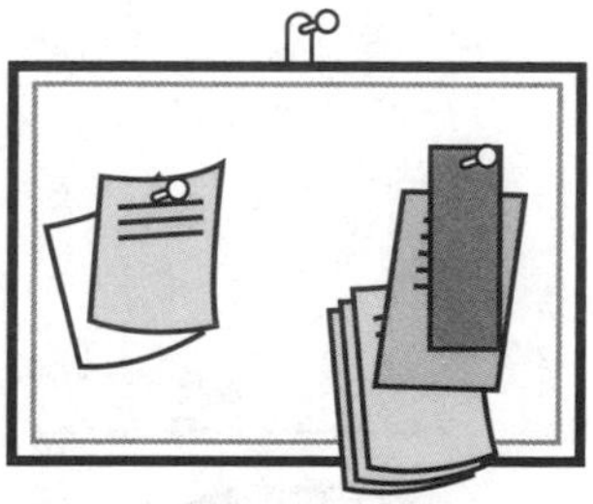

You don't have to spend a lot of money on the party itself. Limit it to a couple of hours. A few snacks such as fruit with yogurt dip, a vegetable platter, chips and dip, and soft drinks or herbal teas is all you need. The purpose is not to feed people a meal, but just to entice them to come in and see your new space (or your newly revitalized space) and to acquaint them with the services you have to offer. Have plenty of your business cards and brochures on hand to pass out.

If you're already in business, you could host a Customer Appreciation Day. Besides having food and drink on hand, you may want to do something else special for your clients. How about asking a chiropractor to attend and do free spinal analysis on people, or ask a nurse to give free blood pressure checks? Be creative. If you have the space, consider asking the Red Cross to conduct a blood drive at your business on that day—and offer everyone who gives a pint of blood a coupon for ten dollars off on a massage.

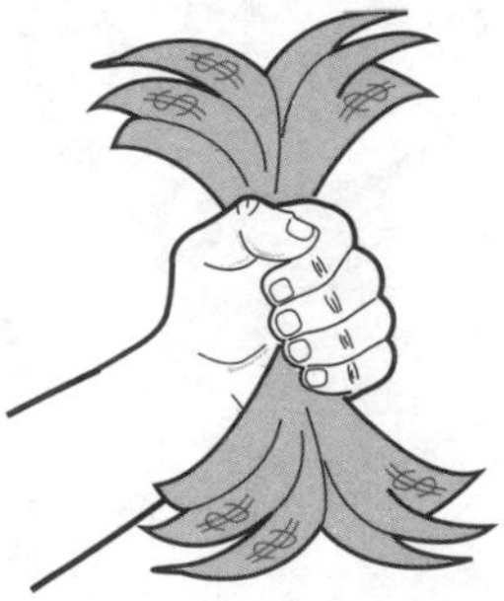

If you've been in business for a while, take a look around your office. If the paint's looking tired, consider doing some redecorating. You can spruce your office up cheaply. Move the furniture around and get a few new plants, hang a new pair of curtains or a new picture in the lobby. Get a nice little water fountain or an unusual lamp. Then invite people in to see your revitalized space and for customer appreciation. Have some giveaways on hand or offer a drawing for a free massage. Offer your existing clients a small free gift for bringing someone to the party that you've never met.

A party is a party! Have some balloons and a banner outside announcing your event. If it's allowable, consider renting a flashing sign for a day to draw in people off the street. Carry the party atmosphere inside by having a nice flower arrangement in the lobby, some lit candles around, and nice soothing music playing in the background. You are showcasing your office in the best possible light.

Another thing to consider for your grand opening is asking a radio station to do a live remote broadcast from your business. Again, the grand opening is the time to spend some money. Depending on the area you live and how populated it is, radio advertising may seem like too much of an expense, but in smaller towns, it's usually affordable. One of our local radio stations will give me a two-hour remote broadcast, during which they guarantee me ten minutes of the airtime to say whatever I want to about the business, ten guaranteed blurbs about the business, and they provide pizza and soft drinks to everyone who comes to the event, for the paltry sum of $300.

Ask a staff member, friend, or spouse to help you with keeping drinks on ice or food replenished during the party so that you personally can meet and greet everyone that comes in.

Other Businesses' Grand Openings

In the course of a year, how many businesses will open that are within close proximity of your office? There will probably be a few, at least. Whenever you see a business getting ready to open, call or stop in to introduce yourself and offer to do free chair massage at *their* grand opening. This is extending a welcome to the new business, helping them make their opening a success, while at the same time providing you with another opportunity to meet new people. You might want to print some discount coupons that say something like "for the customers of Fred's Automotive Shop" to give to attendees. Be sure to have plenty of your business cards and brochures and your sign-up list on hand. You could even take your appointment book along and make appointments right there on the spot. Don't forget to take some gift certificates with you whenever you go out somewhere. You might make a sale!

My Story

Vern's Story

I only do house calls and corporate massage. Since I have no office, a grand opening or open house doesn't personally work for me—but I attend as many as I can within a 20 mile radius of my home. Whenever I see one advertised, I just go to the business a day or two beforehand, introduce myself, and ask if they'd like to have free chair massage at their event. I have never been turned down! I always get a few clients from these events. And, several of the owners of the places I've been have even hired me to come back monthly or quarterly to do chair massage on their employees.

Make it a goal to participate in at least two other grand openings during the year.

My Personal Journey

This Week's Activity: A Grand Opening Date ____________

For this week's activity, you are going to plan your Grand Opening, or plan to participate in one that someone else is having, if you are not in business for yourself. Write down ideas for refreshments, entertainment, health-related activities, free sample massages, a drawing, or whatever you are going to do to make your party a success. If you've already been in business for a while, take the concept and have an anniversary celebration or other type of open house instead.

My Goals

____

____

____

What's in my way?

____

____

____

What action can I take to remedy the situation?

____

____

____

One-Year Progress Update Date ____________

____

____

____

POSITIVE AFFIRMATION: **Every day that my business is open is a grand opening.**

CHAPTER

16

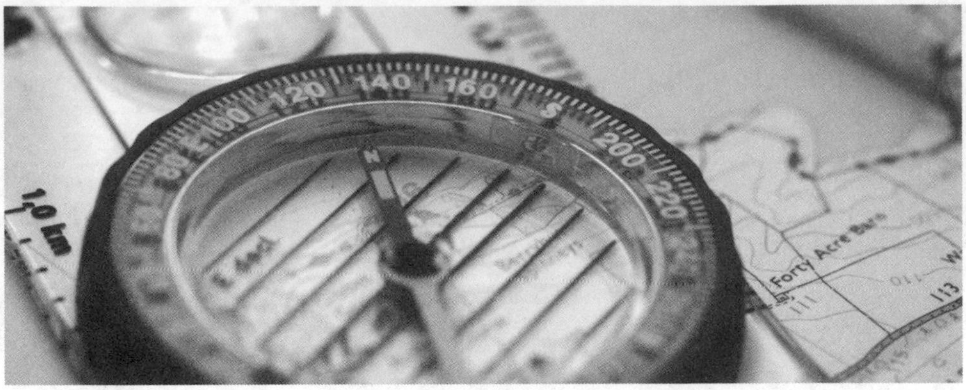

Get Involved in Your Community

STRATEGY is: A style of thinking, a conscious and deliberate process, an intensive implementation system, the science of insuring FUTURE SUCCESS.
—Pete Johnson

Along with performing community service, you simply have to get out in your community and get involved. It may seem like a paradox to say you have to get out of your office in order to get new people into it, but that's true.

Besides the Chamber of Commerce, there are probably dozens of other civic and community groups in your area: the Lions Club, Civitans, Ruritans, the Optimist Club, Sertoma, and so forth. And of course, you can't join every single one. But belonging to one and getting together once a month with a group outside your immediate circle will be beneficial. You'll meet new people and have the opportunity to be involved in worthwhile causes. The groups that you can't personally join are still possible venues for you to publicize yourself, because they are always on the lookout for good speakers. Offer to give a talk on the health benefits of massage, getting rid of stress, or living well with fibromyalgia—that one always works well for me because there are so many people with the diagnosis nowadays (it's probably over-diagnosed, but that's beyond our control).

Communities also tend to have specialized groups that are devoted to local causes, like environmental concerns. In my town, there are currently groups such as "Save The Old Jail" and "Stop Logging." If you choose to get involved in a group that is devoted to a controversial cause, don't be surprised if the fallout comes to the front door of your business. If you make it to the front page of the newspaper looking angry and holding a sign that says "Down with logging," then you can expect that no loggers will be patronizing your business. Follow your conscience, of course, but keep in mind that as a business person, you don't want to alienate the public, even a small faction of it.

Town meetings are open to the public. Not only are local elected officials in attendance, but usually so are other trades people who want to keep abreast of what's going on in case it should have any effect on them and their business. Again, it's a good opportunity to meet people, and it's also smart business to know what's going on at the local government level. As there is usually a period of time when the public is allowed to speak, it's a chance to make your opinion heard as well.

If you live in a large city, your ability to meet and greet may be confined to a few blocks radius. If you live in a small town, make the resolution that you will visit every business on Main Street during the year. Take a stack of business cards and go into every store or other business. Introduce yourself. In small towns, merchants tend to support the people who support them. When you have a need for something, try to shop in town instead of going down the bypass to the big superstore—unless your office is located next to the superstore. In that case, by all means, cultivate the employees and others there as clients, but if you're in town, support those small business people. After all, *you* have a small business and you want *them* to support *you*.

Lisa's Story

My Story

When I graduated from massage school, I wanted to work at the nicest spa in our town, which is on Main Street. I approached the owner and told her I would be willing to sit there and take walk-in clients since their regular therapists were usually booked up. I didn't sit, though. I would just take a handful of brochures and go up and down the street introducing myself to the store owners and even people on the street, and talk to them about massage. Within a month I had as many clients as the regulars, and the owner was getting another new graduate to "sit around." I didn't wait for my clients to come in the door. I dragged them in!

As stated in Chapter 6, consider everyone in your community as a potential client. The more of them you meet, the more of them you have the opportunity to expose your business to. Your fellow merchants, your church family, the people you see at the grocery store are all potential clients—but they may not know it if you don't tell them! You might run into the same people at the bank every Friday when you go in to make a deposit. You nod and smile at each other. Take that further—hand them a business card and introduce yourself. Be proactive. Remember that you are on a mission to increase the amount of people you know and who know about your business.

My husband and I are members of the Loyal Order of the Moose—commonly referred to as the Moose Lodge. The Moose supports some wonderful causes such as children's homes. This is one of those great organizations that has the policy that if you are a member of one, you are a member of all, so in spite of the fact that we live in North Carolina, we can walk into any Moose Lodge in the world and be welcomed with open arms. An organization like that is a great thing for people who move to a new town—to have a ready-made group you can join right in with. We have visited Moose Lodges across the country while traveling, and we have been made to feel genuinely welcome in every single one. Our lodge has several raffles throughout the year, and I usually donate a free massage. One of those winners has purchased gift certificates for at least a half-dozen family members and has recommended us to many more. It is one of those instances of giving a little and getting a lot in return.

You don't necessarily have to limit yourself to civic organizations. Garden clubs, book clubs, nature clubs, diet groups, and so on are other possibilities. Make it a part of your one-year plan to join at least one civic or social club or attend at least one of their functions per month. Now go forth and meet people!

My Personal Journey

This Week's Activity: Getting Involved in My Community Date ____________

For this week's activity, you are going to make an effort to be involved in your community. Join at least one civic organization or club that you are not a member of and be a proactive member. If you previously belonged to another group that you haven't been active in for a while, renew that relationship. Visit at least two other businesses near you that you have never been into and introduce yourself and tell them about your business. Attend at least one community function, whether that's a town meeting or church social, and make it a point to talk to at least three people about your business. Remember to be armed with business cards and brochures.

My Goals

___

___

___

What's in my way?

___

___

___

What action can I take to remedy the situation?

___

___

___

One-Year Progress Update Date ____________

___

___

___

POSITIVE AFFIRMATION: **I am a vital part of my community.**

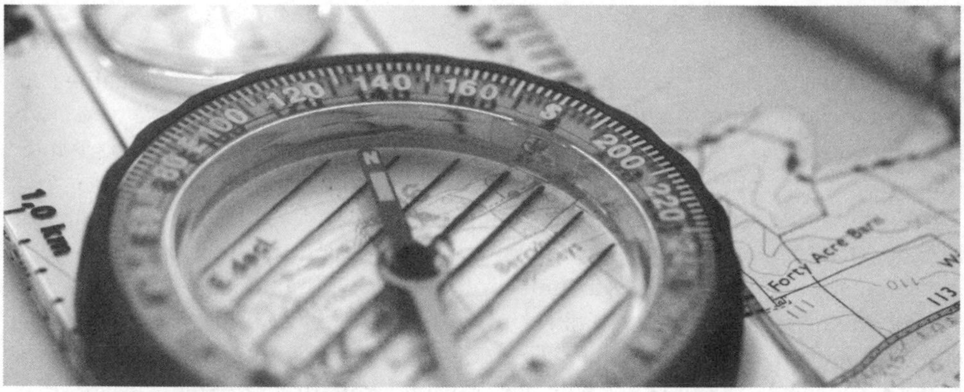

CHAPTER 17

Community Service

Success is not the key to happiness. Happiness is the key to success. If you love what you are doing, you will be successful.

—Herman Cain

Remember this: the more you give it away, the more it will come back to you. Community service can come in many forms.

The American Massage Therapy Association (AMTA) has Emergency Response Massage Teams in most states and in many foreign countries. I'm a member of our state chapter. Wherever there's a disaster, team members volunteer their time to go and massage emergency responders. When the World Trade Center was destroyed, massage teams from all over the country came to massage the firefighters, police officers, and other emergency personnel on the scene. These great teams go wherever there are tornadoes, hurricanes, or other devastating weather, and any place where a traumatic event requiring emergency response has occurred.

Beckie's Story

I do for a living what most therapists do for community service—I work full-time in a hospice. I started out there as a nurse's aide and the director approached me about attending massage school, and the company actually paid my tuition in exchange for the promise that I would work there at least two years after graduation. I massage both the patients and the staff in exchange for my pay. In addition, in my off time I can massage family members who are visiting the hospice, which I do at a discounted rate. I make it a point to get out of the hospice at least one day per month to do community service in some other setting. My two year commitment to them is up now, and I don't want to leave the hospice, but I have found it is important for me to get out and work in other environments to keep from getting burned out.

My Story

Community service may mean volunteering time at a hospice, massaging staff members who perform such a difficult job, or bringing comfort to those who are in their last days and hours. Community service may mean doing free or discounted massage on someone you know who truly needs it and can't afford it.

Community service may mean doing free massage at health fairs, church socials, street festivals, and anywhere else they'll let you set up a chair or table.

Community service serves a number of purposes. First, it is a way to give back something to your community. It may be your tithe. Second, it is a way to make your presence known in the community. The more your name and face are out there, the better off you are. If your office happens to be on Main Street in Small Town, USA, most people probably know you are there. If your office isn't as visible as that, some people probably don't know that you (and your services) exist.

Prepare to Publicize

When performing community service, always go prepared with plenty of business cards, brochures, menu of services, or any other literature pertaining to your business. If you plan to do a lot of outdoor events, a tent is a nice investment that doesn't cost much. I purchased one that comfortably houses a table for my literature, a massage table, and a massage chair for around fifty dollars. A custom printed banner with your name on it is another inexpensive investment, and computer-savvy individuals may even be able to print one out on their own.

Particularly at street fairs or other events that are open to the public, community service is always a photo opportunity. My staff members and I have been photographed by our local newspaper many times while performing massage at community events, and enjoyed the benefit of seeing our picture in the newspaper (along with the line identifying our business) absolutely free.

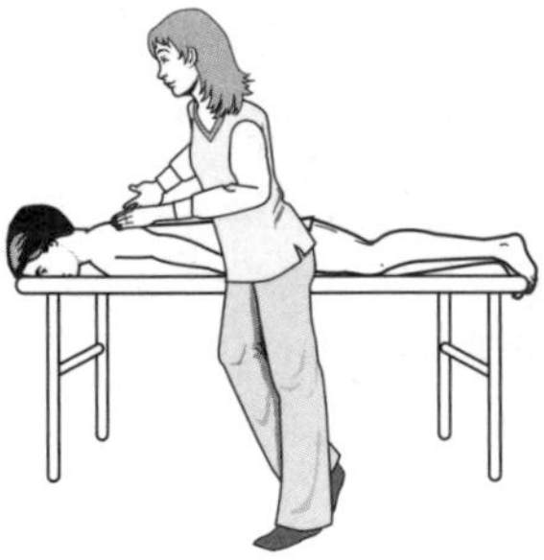

Choosing Wisely

Community service is an opportunity to be in service, to educate the public about massage, and an opportunity to meet potential new clients. Having said that, choose your community service selectively. You can't say yes to everyone who calls on you; otherwise, you'd never have time to run your business and make money. You may need to set a limit as our clinic has, on how many events we can do per month, or what days we can be available. If Monday is the slowest day in your office, that may be the day you designate as your community service day. If someone calls on you, you can always explain that you will be glad to massage the nurses at the local free clinic for Nurse's Appreciation Week, as long as you could come on Monday. Most of us can't afford to give up our busiest day of the week to do free massage at community events.

In the same vein, you may get many requests for gift certificates donated to this event or that cause. You may need to set a policy regarding how many and of what value you can afford to give away within a year. One good idea is to only give away gift certificates that are good for a half hour of massage, and print right on them that the massage can be upgraded to an hour for just $25, or whatever you'd like to charge. It's been my experience that about half the recipients will go for the upgrade.

Incidentally, giving away gift certificates has a couple of advantages over actually going somewhere to do free massage. First, you don't have to lose appointments by being away from your office. The recipient will come to you. Second, and this is almost unbelievable—but some people will never redeem those certificates, and you won't be out anything at all, but you'll still have the good will you generated when you gave it to the event or charity to start with. Third, people who win a prize of any kind, even a gift certificate, are usually so thrilled that they tell people about it—a little word of mouth advertising. Fourth, after they come to redeem the certificate and find out what an awesome therapist you are, they'll talk about that too. Word of mouth is the cheapest advertising you can have.

While one of the purposes of community service is to give to the community, that doesn't mean your primary purpose of making a living has to go by the wayside while you're doing it. Choose your community service events selectively with the intention that they will generate a payoff for you in the future. At least one or two of those grateful nurses you massage during Nurse's Appreciation Week are going to make appointments and become clients. The same with street fairs and bigger events—whenever you are exposing yourself to a larger number of people, there is a larger number of potential clients.

This is not to say you can't give away massage without expecting anything in return. You should give it to any person, event, or organization that tugs at your personal heartstrings if you feel led to do so. But if you choose to also utilize community service as a marketing tool, and you know you can only do a certain amount of it, be wise about it. Here are two examples of poor choices:

A therapist I know gave every contestant in our county's junior miss pageant a gift certificate for a free massage. There were 18 young ladies around age 16–18, who are spending their discretionary money on clothes, their car, the latest in electronic gadgetry, and their boyfriends. They came to get their free massage, and never came back. Most moved away to college. There wasn't a good candidate for return clients in the whole bunch, and there is 18 hours of massage the therapist gave up, around a thousand dollars at her prices. That's a nice weekend at the beach.

A merchant in town who has never been a client here, but owns a business that I occasionally patronize, called and wanted volunteers to come to her daughter's Girl Scout campout. The campout was in a state park almost 50 miles away, the request was to massage Girl Scouts who were from 8 to 10 years old, and with the exception of her own daughter and a couple more, most of the girls were from other towns. We had to decline that one. It was on Saturday, a busy day in our office, and there was little potential for return. If—and it's a big if—if the person who had made that request was a regular, long-standing client who has sent me many referrals over the years, I would have been more inclined to honor that request. Or maybe I could have helped her by calling a massage school near the camping area to see if they could send students to do the massage. It depends on how accommodating you want to be.

Points to Consider

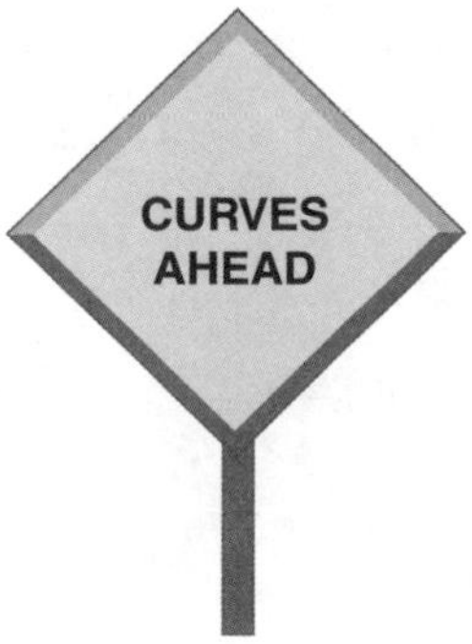

When you make a choice to give someone free or discounted massage based on their need and your own benevolence, examine your own feelings carefully before jumping in. Be sure that you can spare the time—and the money—before you decide to replace a paying appointment with a non-paid one. Be certain you won't come to regret it or become resentful about the time you are giving up.

People sometimes tend not to value things very much when they're free. There are, of course, exceptions, but I observed one incidence of this with another friend who's a therapist. My friend felt sorry for a client who was going through a bitter and expensive divorce and the woman could no longer afford her weekly massages. She had always been a client who tended to run late for her appointments, but prior to the nasty divorce proceedings had also been a very generous tipper to make up for it. When the therapist continued to give her massage for a couple of months, she continued her pattern of being chronically late, only now she was neither paying for the session nor tipping at all. It quickly became a thorn in the therapist's side and was a no-win situation for everyone when the therapist finally had to cut her off, with resentment on all sides.

Performing community service by giving away massage to deserving individuals gives you a warm, fuzzy feeling when it's the right thing to do, but consider that having some sort of energy exchange also allows the client to maintain their dignity. Maybe vegetables from their garden or babysitting your child, or asking them to answer the phone in your office for an hour or two so you can run errands or have time off is a better solution than outright giving it away in some cases. You will still be generating good will, and the recipient will still tell people what a wonderful therapist and person you are.

Some business and marketing books deride community service and make it sound like a crime to give away your services. I say that is hogwash. Give with willing hands and a willing heart, and you shall receive many benefits, both personal and financial. If you're a licensed professional, the massage you give away may even be a tax deduction for you. Check with your tax professional.

My Personal Journey

This Week's Activity: Performing Community Service Date ____________

For this week's activity, you are going to perform, or at least schedule, several opportunities for community service. If you are still a student, you may be obligated to perform a certain number of hours of community service before you can graduate. Even if this is not the case and you're an old hand at massage, get out into the community and massage some deserving individuals without compensation, just to publicize your business and to renew yourself.

My Goals

____

____

____

What's in my way?

____

____

____

What action can I take to remedy the situation?

____

____

____

One-Year Progress Update Date ____________

____

____

____

POSITIVE AFFIRMATION: **Serving the community nourishes me.**

CHAPTER

18

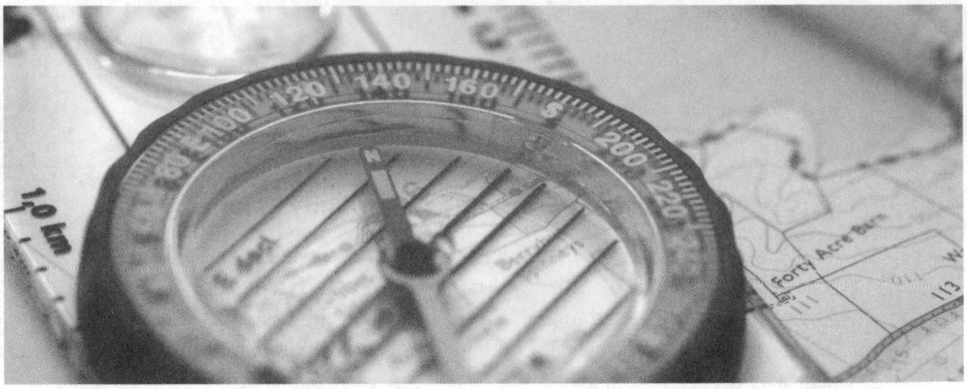

Mutual Referral Relationships

The road to success leads through the valley of humility, and the path is up the ladder of patience and across the wide barren plains of perseverance. As yet, no short cut has been discovered.

—Joseph J. Lamb

Mutual referral relationships can be a huge source of income. You will want to cultivate mutual referrals with therapists who have different specialties than yours, therapists who keep different days or hours than yours, and therapists who live in other towns. I know therapists from all over the state due to my teaching and involvement in AMTA. When a tourist passing through tells me they live at the coast, for instance, I can usually recommend someone in their area. People are very appreciative of those gestures.

My Story

Barb's Story

I live and practice near a military base, which means my clients are sometimes short-term due to their being assigned somewhere else. When someone tells me they're moving, I always take the time to look on my professional association's website and find them a therapist in the area they're moving to. I have had calls and thank-you notes from therapists all over, and from the clients themselves, thanking me for doing this for them. Especially when people move to a state that may not have licensure, the clients are grateful to know they are going to a reputable and professional person.

I choose not to have any nail services in my office, because I don't want the chemical smell in the air. But I know other therapists who do have that service, so when people call and ask for that, I'll refer them. The particular therapist nearest me who does have that service available does not do any deep tissue work; she is strictly a Swedish practitioner, and she in turn sends her people who want or need deep work to my office. I may lose an occasional client who decides it's more convenient to get their nails done and their massage in one stop, but it's more than made up for by the pain and injury clients she sends my way.

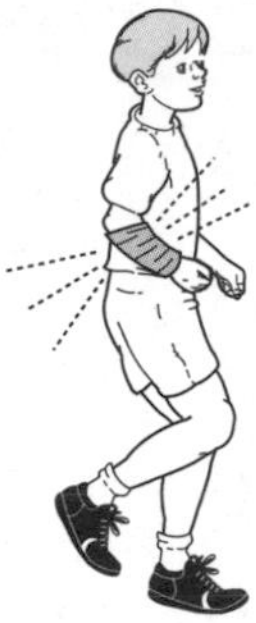

Physicians

Doctors, for the most part, are a hard nut to crack. However, if you search diligently, you can probably find at least a few physicians in your area who will acknowledge the efficacy of massage in treating numerous conditions. AMTA has posters available that are all about the medical benefits of massage for therapists to present to physicians. Some physicians, like some members of the general public, still have the massage = sex picture in their mind, or they think it's fluff and puff for ladies who lunch, and it is up to you to change their mind. If you are only practicing relaxation massage, it may be more difficult for you to cultivate doctors, but it can still be done. So many conditions people suffer from are all about stress, and an hour of good Swedish massage can make a big difference to them and their well-being. If you are a medically oriented massage therapist, you will have a much wider physician audience.

I have a letter that I send out to doctors that I'll include at the end of this section. Write something similar for yourself, and send it to every doctor in your area. I don't overlook any specialty. Every doctor has clients with stress-related conditions. General practitioners have people suffering everything from a headache to repetitive motion injuries to broken bones—all things we can help in the recovery of. Dentists are a major source of referrals at my office for TMJ work. Let me share with you the value of getting client testimonials on that front.

A woman who is a receptionist in a dentist's office near mine was on the table getting a Swedish massage when she mentioned how her TMJ was bothering her. Her employer had already given her an appliance to wear at night because she was grinding her teeth. I persuaded her to let me do a TMJ sequence on her. She experienced immediate relief, and of course went back and told the dentist. I sent him a letter of introduction. He referred another client almost immediately.

The woman he referred was treated by another therapist in my office. This lady was so thrilled with the results, that without any prompting whatsoever, she wrote a letter to the editor of the newspaper thanking the therapist and praising the doctor. Her letter said something similar to, "Thanks to Dr. Miller for not being too proud to send me to Carla at THERA-SSAGE. He could have fitted me with an appliance, given me drugs, or recommended surgery, but instead, he cared more about me than he did about his pocketbook." What a chain reaction that set off! The week that appeared in the paper, we probably got 20 calls for TMJ work. I sent the dentist a nice thank-you card. That is the kind of positive publicity that neither he nor I could buy with all the money in the world.

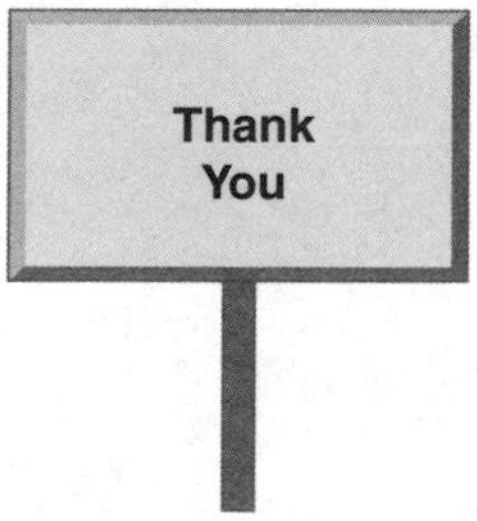

It is very important, if you cultivate doctor referrals, that you follow up with them for each and every client they send you. I send a thank-you note and always state that we will be sending progress notes—and we do. I just say something like,

> Dear Dr. Miller,
>
> Thank you for your referral of Rose Jones to our office for TMJ work. We have scheduled her for three visits and will send you the progress notes at the end of her treatment. We appreciate your confidence in our services.
>
> Sincerely,
> Laura Allen, LMBT

Don't fail to follow up! The doctor may receive solicitations from other therapists, and he will undoubtedly stick with the one who is the most professional and communicative.

Sample Physician's Letter

Laura Allen, LMBT
THERA-SSAGE
431 S. Main St., Ste. 2
Rutherfordton, NC 28139

Dr. John Smith
500 Main St.
Rutherfordton, NC 28139

June 1, 2006

Dear Dr. Smith,

I would like to introduce you to the services offered at THERA-SSAGE. Our office is staffed by massage therapists and bodyworkers who are all North Carolina licensed and Nationally Certified. You may not be familiar with all the benefits of massage therapy and how it can help your patients. I have enclosed a brochure for you, "The Benefits of Massage."

Our staff members have extensive training in treating stress-related conditions, repetitive motion injuries such as carpal tunnel syndrome, athletic injuries, chronic conditions such as fibromyalgia, TMJ dysfunction, migraine headaches, and many more conditions.

Massage is noninvasive. We can effect pain relief and rehabilitation, help restore lost range of motion and flexibility, and relieve the stress that is the root cause of so many conditions.

We would be very grateful to receive any referrals from you that you might send our way. We will update you regularly with progress notes for anyone that you refer to us. I would like to invite you to stop by our office to see our facility and meet our staff members at your convenience. Please give us a call at 288-3727 to let us know when you can come by.

Enclosed are a few of our business cards. Please remind any clients you might send our way to let us know that they were referred by you. If you would like more information about massage, or would like some testimonials and/or references from existing clients, please don't hesitate to call on us. Our office does accept insurance. I know that will matter to some of your patients.

Thanks so much for your consideration.

Sincerely,
Laura Allen, LMBT

Chiropractors

Chiropractors are my biggest source of mutual referrals. My staff members and I have cultivated relationships with a number of chiropractors all over our county. For one thing, most of us personally visit chiropractors ourselves, and we don't all see the same one. For another thing, most of the chiropractors in our area have awakened to the fact that people need massage along with chiropractic in order for their own work to go more efficiently and for the results to last longer. They realize that shortened muscles are responsible for pulling bones out of alignment and they know that massage can lengthen the muscle back to normal.

Rather than endorsing just one particular chiropractor, I occasionally print an article about chiropractic, and how massage is a great complement to it in my newsletter along with the numbers of a half-dozen practitioners, and encourage people to see the one most conveniently located to them. That way I don't alienate anyone of them. We make sure that they're all stocked with some of our business cards on a regular basis. We also call their office to tell them that we have referred so-and-so to them and make the first appointment for the client while the client is standing right there in our office. That's a courtesy to them and the client.

While massage therapists are not supposed to prescribe or diagnose, the fact is that many times while standing over someone's back during a massage, we can often spot obvious misalignments or other problems that we know would benefit from chiropractic, and shouldn't hesitate to suggest it when called for; don't overstep your boundaries as a massage therapist. Just say, "You look like you may have a misalignment going on; you might benefit from a visit to the chiropractor." Do not say "Your T-4 and -5 is out. You need to go to the chiropractor." That's diagnosing, which is clearly outside the scope of our practice.

As with physicians, be sure to thank the chiropractor and send progress notes as a follow-up.

Mental Health Professionals

Occasionally, we're all confronted with a client who needs something we can't provide—mental health (assuming you're not a psychologist in addition to being a massage therapist). It's not in our scope of practice to provide counseling to people. Each quarter when our state massage board sends out their newsletter, there are almost always reports of a therapist being sanctioned for providing services they are not qualified to provide, and nine times out of ten, it's because a therapist was trying to act as a counselor. Leave that to the people who have the proper training. People do tend sometimes to tell us their problems. That doesn't mean for you to get embroiled in them, and it certainly doesn't mean to give them advice.

The main reason I personally refer anyone is usually depression. People with fibromyalgia and other chronic pain conditions are depressed! Depression and illness feed off each other. If you're ill, you're depressed about it, and the more depressed you are, the more likely you are to become ill. Stress attacks whatever part of the body is most vulnerable. You can't come out and tell someone rudely that you think they need to see a shrink. You have to handle it with tact and diplomacy. I can say, "You know, one of my other clients with fibro became so depressed, she started seeing Dr. Feelgood for counseling, and she says she feels a hundred times better. I've got his number if you'd like to check him out." I certainly don't want to encourage people to go on drugs, but depression is sometimes just a chemical imbalance in the brain that can be helped by drug therapy. So far, no one has gotten mad at me for making the suggestion that they might want to seek help.

Acupuncturists, Naturopaths, and Other Alternative Practitioners

Many massage therapists—probably the majority—are into natural means of treating illness. Complementary and alternative medicine (CAM) is wellness-based medicine, as opposed to the sickness-based kind we have all been exposed to. If you have relationships with other practitioners of the natural kind of healing arts, they are also good sources of mutual referrals. Because of the sickness-based paradigm of medicine that most people have grown up with, people may be hesitant to visit a CAM practitioner. I would never pressure anyone to go where they don't feel comfortable. On the other hand, I always point out that natural medicine is noninvasive, usually very reasonable in price compared to prescription drugs, and has no harmful side effects, which in itself is enough to impress most people. It goes without saying that you never tell anyone to quit taking their prescription drugs or advise them to dump their oncologist to seek a natural cure for cancer. But do keep the business cards of other practitioners on hand for referral purposes. Allow the client to make up his own mind without any coercing from you.

Personal Trainers

One of my most lucrative mutual relationships is with a personal trainer. During the average week, we send each other anywhere from one to a half-dozen clients. He first approached me about buying gift certificates to give to his clients who had met their weight-loss goals. I ended up being his client, he ended up being mine, and it mushroomed from there. In the past two years, he has probably referred 50 or 60 people to me, and vice versa. I display his literature in my office, and he displays mine in his gym. He carries my cards all the time. I carry his. When someone says, "You look like you've lost weight," I whip out one of his cards and give it to them. It's a great relationship. You may not need to lose weight, but surely you have clients who do, and cultivating a relationship with a personal trainer is a great marketing strategy for both of you. Look at how many of your clients need to exercise. And he has clients who have injured themselves or just need stress relief. It's a "win-win" situation for you, for the trainer, and for the client.

All Your Clients

Your clients are the best source of referrals you are ever going to have. The first client I ever had sent the second. The second sent the third. It snowballed from there. When you get a new client, always ask them how they heard about your business, and be sure to thank the client who sent them, whether that's by some sort of client reward (more about that in Chapter 23) or just a thank-you by way of a phone call or personal note.

My Personal Journey

This Week's Activity: Cultivating Mutual Referral Relationships

Date ____________________

For this week's activity, you are going to start cultivating mutual referral relationships, or revitalize old ones that you may already have if you're a licensed practitioner. Make a list of doctors, dentists, other massage therapists, mental health professionals, and other health care professionals, both traditional and alternative/complementary, that you can refer to who would be willing to refer to you. Make personal contact whenever possible; write a professional-sounding letter introducing yourself and your services whenever you can't see the practitioner in person. When going to meet people you may cultivate a referral relationship with, be sure to have plenty of your business cards to leave with them. It's also nice of you to provide your own card holder.

My Goals

____

____

____

What's in my way?

____

____

____

What action can I take to remedy the situation?

____

____

____

One-Year Progress Update

Date ____________________

____

____

____

POSITIVE AFFIRMATION: **I graciously and appreciatively give and receive referrals.**

CHAPTER

19

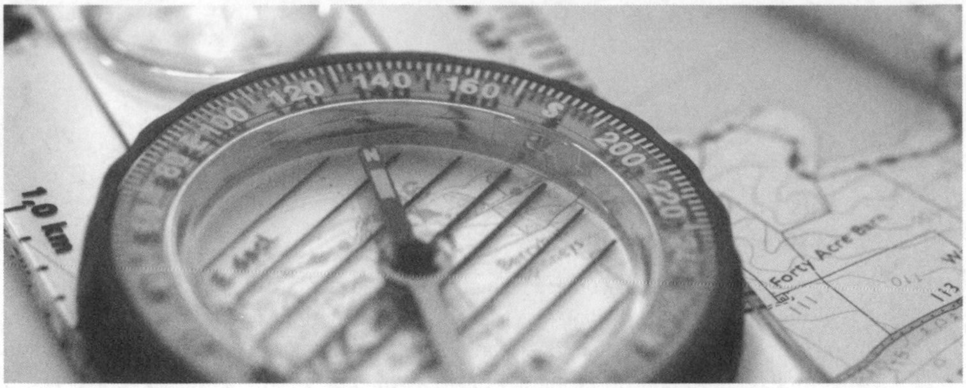

Partners in Advertising

Success is a science; if you have the conditions, you get the result.
—Oscar Wilde

While it's true we want the majority of our energy focused on no-cost and low-cost marketing, spending dollars on advertising is a reality for most of us. You can cut that cost by using the "Partners in Advertising" method. These partners can be everything from suppliers to chiropractors to other therapists.

Splitting the Cost

Two friends of mine, both therapists, live and have their offices in opposite ends of our county—separated by 30 or so miles. They share a centrally located highway billboard that neither could afford by themselves. If you have a mutual referral relationship with a chiropractor or other health care practitioner, he/she may be a good candidate for sharing advertising. That is exponentially so if they are located in the same building—you could share costs on everything from radio ads to signage to printed materials.

My Story

Carol's Story

I probably get the most new customers from the free advertising that local realtors do for me. I have several realtors who are loyal customers, and they have the opportunity to meet a lot of new people moving into the area. They all keep a supply of my business cards. I reward them by giving them an occasional free massage or a gift certificate to a nice restaurant.

Approach the other therapists in your area, and ask them to contribute to a full-page ad for Massage Therapy Awareness Week, or during holidays, for instance, to get a high-impact ad at a low cost for everyone. A full-page ad may be

$1,000, but if ten therapists chip in, that's $100 each, much more affordable, and everybody wins.

Getting Other People to Promote Your Business

Partners in advertising also applies to places that will let you display your cards or brochures and you would do the same for them. Don't overlook any possibilities. You, of course, want to have your literature displayed in the offices of people you have mutual referral relationships with (and theirs on display in your office), but there are many other possibilities.

Do you have any clients who are in the real estate business? Suggest to them that purchasing a gift certificate for a client who has just bought property from them is a nice thank you gesture—and that if they purchase a package deal of these from you, they'll get them at a discounted price. This has worked for me with a lot of realtors. Another tactic is to print business-size discount cards—just do it yourself on your computer—that have the realtor's name on them so you'll know where they came from. Mine look like this:

> You must be a VIP, if you're with
> **Alice Jones of Ajax Realty**
> This card entitles you to $10 off your
> first massage at THERA-SSAGE
> 431 S. Main St., Rutherfordton, NC
> 288-3727

The realtors appreciate these cards—after all, they're not costing them anything, but it's a gift they can give to clients and potential clients. You'll get results from these cards for several reasons. People buying real estate are often transplants who are just moving into your town. They don't have a massage therapist yet. Others may be people who are natives just moving into your neighborhood, and it may be more convenient for them to come to you than to drive 50 miles to see their old therapist. If it's someone who is purchasing commercial real estate, there may be a new business for you to partner with or to approach for corporate massage opportunities. People who have the money to purchase real estate probably have the money to spend on massage.

Cards like the one above also work great for other service businesses. Entice the realtors or other business people by offering them the discount or an occasional free massage—say when ten of their cards have been turned in. People pick up dry cleaning every day. Plumbers, carpet cleaners, and maid services are out in people's homes every day. Beauticians are with the public all day long. There's no end to the realm of possible partners

Opportunities are everywhere. I recently read a tip on the Internet from a therapist whose office happened to be near a take-out pizza parlor. She approached the manager and asked if he would be willing to put discount coupons in the pizza boxes, and the answer was yes! Immediately, each day, dozens of her coupons started going out. In just two weeks she had booked twenty new clients. This tactic will work in any restaurant that does takeout meals. When you make your coupon proposal to the manager, always point out that it appears that his business is doing something nice for the customers by offering the discount coupons—people may even get the

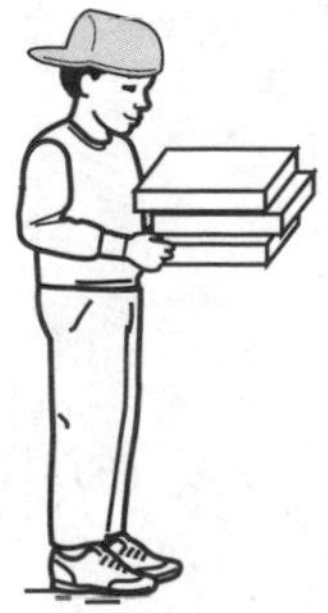

impression that the business is subsidizing the coupons. Bakeries, coffee shops, sub shops, even full-service restaurants are possible venues for this plan.

This is not a one-way street. When people send business your way, it's nice if you send it their way as well. Those folks just moving into town are going to need a plumber or a maid service someday. When people agree to hand out my cards, I ask for a supply of theirs. I keep these in an alphabetized card file at the office, and whenever some newcomer asks, "Can you tell me the name of a good caterer?," for instance, I'm able to hand them the card. And I always write on the back, "tell them Laura Allen sent you." That way, the people who are publicizing my business for me are assured that I am also publicizing theirs. I even make it a point to mention to people who tell me they have just moved here that I've lived here for a long time, and that if there's anything I could tell them about the area, or recommend a service person, I'll be glad to, and newcomers appreciate that gesture. It's a "win-win" situation for you, your advertising partners, and the customers of both you and them.

Make it a goal to add a new partner in advertising every month during the year.

My Personal Journey

This Week's Activity: Partnering in Advertising Date ____________

For this week's activity, start cultivating some partners in advertising. These could be other complementary businesses, such as chiropractic offices or other alternative health care practitioners. Research the cost of billboards in your area to see if it would be financially feasible for you to share one with someone. Make a list of other possible ways to partner with others to the advantage of both parties and possible venues for doing just that. Take advantage of every opportunity can find to partner in advertising.

My Goals

____

____

____

What's in my way?

____

____

____

What action can I take to remedy the situation?

____

____

____

One-Year Progress Update Date ____________

____

____

____

POSITIVE AFFIRMATION: **Partnering with others is a positive experience for me and for them.**

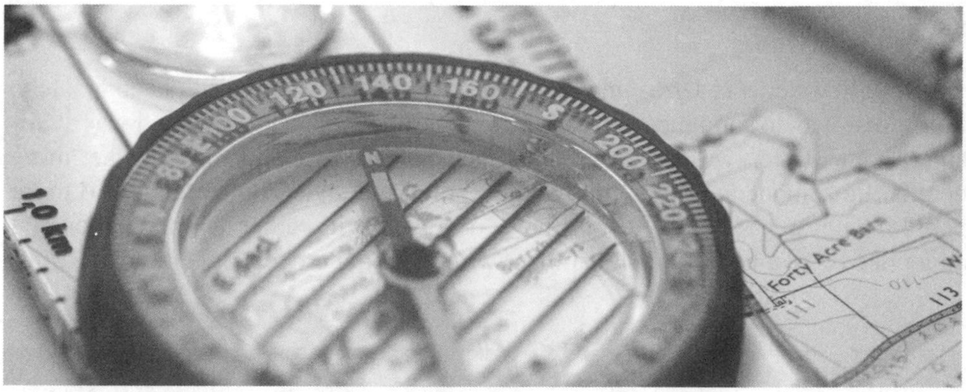

CHAPTER 20

Publishing a Newsletter

Many of life's failures are people who did not realize how close they were to success when they gave up.

—Calvin Coolidge

A newsletter for your business serves several purposes. It keeps you in touch with existing clients, and it can be used to bring in new ones as well. Several companies that cater to the massage trade offer ready-made newsletters that you can personalize to some extent, or you may opt to create your own like I do.

I sent out my first newsletter a few months after I opened my business, and I continue to send them out quarterly. It is one of the most effective marketing tools I have. In addition to sending it out to my clients, I also take copies to community service events, street festivals, the offices of chiropractors and other health professionals I have mutual referral relationships with, and other networking opportunities such as club meetings. I also post it on my website and keep an archive of past issues on the website as well.

My clients know I love to laugh, and I have made humor a big part of the newsletter. Every issue contains a paragraph about "Silly Holidays"—the same silly holidays we talked about in Chapter 2. That's my "hook." You can have your own interesting "hook" (or feel free to use mine). Each issue, I print the silly holidays, which I gathered from the Internet for that quarter, days like "Cow Appreciation Day," "Stop Being Miserable Day," and so forth. People actually called to complain when I left them out one time.

The newsletters which are preprinted usually contain articles about the benefits of massage, a research article or survey, reminders to clients to buy gift certificates, and other features in a similar vein. You can include the same if you decide to write your own, or be as creative as you want to. One of the features of my newsletter is to tell people what my staff and I have been doing—the community service events we're working, the Continuing Education classes we're taking, the therapists who have moved away or gotten married, new staff members and their specialties, and so forth. If you do decide to print your own instead of purchasing a preprinted version, be sure it looks professional. Proofread it, use the spellchecker, be sure the margins look equal, and so forth. Sending one out that looks like a mess is a lot worse than not sending one at all.

Your newsletter is a great memory jogger for clients who haven't been in lately. It's a great way to announce new services. When I announced that Reiki was available at our office, two people who had never heard of Reiki called to get more details, both made appointments, and one of those ended up sending two more people. The same instant results have occurred with other announcements. I announced a two-hour workshop on a raw food diet and twenty people came.

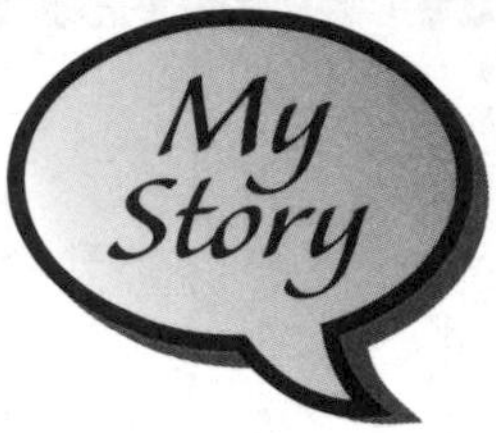

> **_Forrest's Story_**
>
> I send out a newsletter about every two to three months. I purchase them preprinted from a massage supply company, and they come with a blank space for me to personalize them. I use the white space to list my monthly specials, and write about Continuing Ed classes I've taken so clients will know I'm adding to my skills. Sometimes, I order the newsletters that have discount coupons printed on them. My clients always mention that they've received it and seem to appreciate them, so it's worth the money to send them out. Sometimes people who haven't been in lately will call and make an appointment right after they've received it. I think it just jogs their memory that they haven't had a massage in a while.

You can even print discount coupons right on the newsletter. Another therapist I know printed the back of his holiday newsletter with three gift certificates and instructions to call and validate the certificates by giving a credit card number or mailing in a check. He had a blank number line on the certificate, and when a client called to validate, he assigned them a unique number so he could track the certificates. He sold a lot of certificates that way because people didn't even have to make the effort to come by the office to pick it up—they already had it in their hand.

If you have mutual referral relationships with a chiropractor or other professionals, you could even ask if they would like to have an advertisement on your newsletter to help you offset the cost of it, or offer to put in one for free if he/she will do the same for you in *their* newsletter. You can also save money by e-mailing it to the clients who provide you with their e-mail address. Keep extras in the office to give to new clients on their first visit.

Of course you would need to ask their permission first, but you might consider having a section *about* your clients. Ask for testimonials to include in the newsletter, or print something about newsworthy events that have happened for your clients—graduations, awards they've received, a congratulatory note for a client who has opened a new business, for instance. This can generate a lot of good will in the community. Again, ask permission, but you might want to print winners of a contest you have had—for example, "Mary Smith won the free spa package we gave away at the Octoberfest." This can have another benefit, when you're giving out the newsletter at events or people are picking them up in someone else's office. Some people will patronize your business when they read the announcements and think "Oh, "so and so" goes to that massage therapist. I'll go, too."

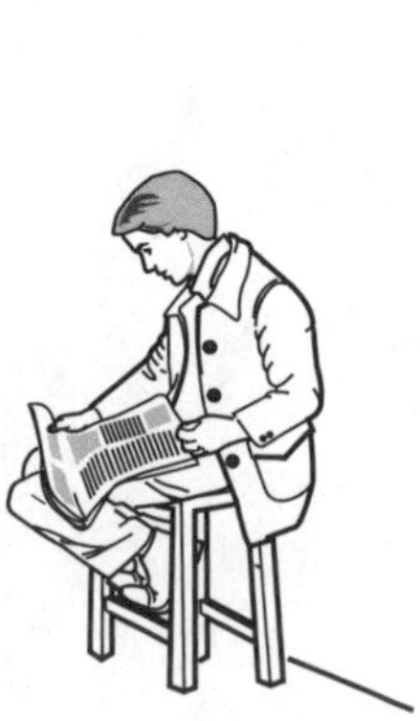

If you run specials, you can include those, too. Since my own newsletter goes out quarterly, I include a section that lists the specials I am running for the next three months. That often has the effect of someone calling in ahead to book a special that's going to be running in the next month or the month after, and spurs people to try services they haven't previously had.

Don't be afraid to toot your own horn, either, if you have had an accomplishment such as a media appearance or winning an award. Your clients would be impressed that you had an article printed in *Massage Magazine*—but people outside the trade don't read it and they won't know if you don't tell them. People will think well of you for volunteering free massages every month to the residents of the abused women's shelter, but again, they won't know if you don't tell them. You're not bragging; you're just spreading a little news, and that's what newsletters are for.

One of my previous newsletters is included below as a sample. Remember, it doesn't have to be fancy—it just has to be interesting and easy to read.

THE THERA-SSAGE TIMES Vol. IX

www.thera-ssage.com 431 S. Main St., Suite 2, Rutherfordton, NC 28139
828-288-3727 therassage@bellsouth.net

If you are new to our business, this is our quarterly newsletter. Thank you for choosing THERA-SSAGE. We know that there are a lot of other places you could go, and we genuinely appreciate your choosing us.

People call to complain if I don't include the "Silly Holidays," so here they are for this quarter: July 10th is "Clerihew Day." The person who sends me the best original clerihew is going to win a free massage. But here's the clincher: It has to be about a public figure. Some of you might have to do a little research to find out what a clerihew is. I'll announce the winner on the website and in the next newsletter. Send your clerihew to our e-mail address therassage@bellsouth.net or send it through snail mail no later than August 30. July 17th is "Cow Appreciation Day." I certainly hope, if you have cows, that you will take a moment to let them know how much you appreciate them. August is "Admit You're Happy Month," so stop trying to act miserable and just be happy. September is "Children's Good Manners Month." Since I'm not a parent, it's easy for me to point the finger. But it does seem kids have a lot less manners these days than when I was a kid. September 15th is "Someday." Remember all those things you are going to do "Someday" and do them today. September 18th is "Wife Appreciation Day." May we recommend a gift certificate from THERA-SSAGE as an appropriate remembrance? September 27th is "Good Neighbor Day." Do something good for your neighbor. They'll be happy and surprised.

THERA-SSAGE hosted a "Meet, Greet and Eat" on July 12th. Around 40 people came out for food and fellowship and to welcome our new staff members, Heather Wiltse, Natalie Veres, and Robert Sunhawk. It was a great evening.

If you aren't a member of the Chamber of Commerce, now's the time to join. And if you are a member, make an effort to participate in more of the functions the Chamber sponsors. "Business After Hours," special classes geared toward small business, networking, and advertising opportunities are just a few of the reasons to be involved.

Laura Earwood Allen, owner of THERA-SSAGE, has finally given birth! It's blue, 8 and ½ × 11 and weighs about a pound. It's the *Plain & Simple Guide to Therapeutic Bodywork & Massage Certification*, and it's already being snapped up by massage schools, according to Lippincott, the publisher. It's available on Lippincott's website at www.lww.com as well as Amazon.com, Barnes & Noble, Waldenbooks, and most massage schools in the United States. We're excited about it.

Lisa Wall is leaving us (again) on August 10th. After staying in Florida for a month while she completed the requirements to get a FL massage license, she is here working while waiting for that important piece of paper to arrive. She'll be living in

Boca Raton and hopefully working at one of those "fancy-schmancy" spas down there. All her regulars be sure to stop in and see her before she's gone for good.

Robert Sunhawk, who works here, is the nephew of the late Chief Two Trees, whom many remember as a gifted healer. On the last weekend of September, there will be a Medicine Moon ceremony and celebration of the life of Chief Two Trees at the Mountain Gateway Museum in Old Fort. This will be Saturday night, September 24th, and Sunday from noon until—with a covered dish dinner Sunday at 4 pm. Robert is collecting stories about the Chief to include in a book. If you had a personal experience with Chief Two Trees, you may send it to us and we will be sure Robert gets it.

We have exciting news that we will talk about again in the next newsletter. THERA-SSAGE has just received permission from the town of Forest City to have a Holistic Health Fair at the Cool Springs Gymnasium on Saturday, October 29 from 9am-3pm. We will be showcasing practitioners from many disciplines of Complementary and Alternative Medicine (CAM). Chiropractic, bodywork of many modalities, acupuncture, aromatherapy, color therapy, sound therapy, light therapy, homeopathy, and naturopathy are just a few of the disciplines we hope to have represented. We are also seeking people who retail items of a holistic therapeutic nature, and organic foods. If you have a skill or product that would fit into this event, please give us a call or e-mail and we will send you the information. This event is nonprofit with proceeds going to the Christmas Cheer Center and Noah's House. Admission to the public will be a donation of a non-perishable food item or toy which will go to the Christmas Cheer Center. Come on out and learn about holistic health care. We want the public to know that there are healthy alternatives to just blindly taking a pill for whatever ails you. If you have been curious about alternative health care, here's your chance to learn about it and support worthwhile charities at the same time. Rutherford Hospital will be there to check blood pressures. If this is successful, and we know it will be, we hope to make it an annual event. Please put that date on your calendar—October 29th. We thank Jimmy Gibson, the mayor of Forest City, the famous and talented Danielle Withrow, and the town council for supporting this event.

I can't say more right now, but we are on the edge of an expansion. An aesthetician will soon be joining our staff and we will be offering a full line of facials, waxing, etc. Be on the lookout in the newspaper and the "Amazin' Shopper." We will definitely advertise the details.

Here are some words of wisdom from Abraham Lincoln (whom we all know was born in Rutherford County):

When I do good, I feel good. When I do bad, I feel bad. That's my religion.

My Personal Journey

This Week's Activity: Publishing a Newsletter Date ____________

For this week's activity, create your own newsletter. If you're still a student, you can create one that tells people about some of your experiences in massage school, when you are going to finish, and what your future work plans are. Go ahead! Send it out to potential clients—friends, family members, people you've met doing practice massages. If you're established, but haven't yet done a newsletter, it's past time for you to do one and send it to all your clients—and anyone you'd like to have as a client.

My Goals

____

____

____

What's in my way?

____

____

____

What action can I take to remedy the situation?

____

____

____

One-Year Progress Update Date ____________

____

____

____

POSITIVE AFFIRMATION: **The news about my business is always positive.**

CHAPTER

21

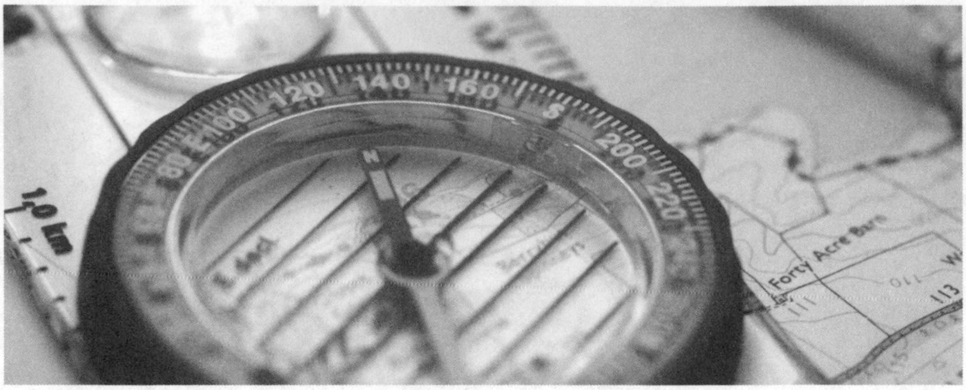

Inexpensive Advertising on the Radio

Every success is built on the ability to do better than good enough.

—Author Unknown

Radio advertising tends to be expensive, especially at the big metropolitan stations, and they usually want you to purchase monthly packages that are beyond the budget of most therapists starting out. When I first started my business, and received a coupon for 50% off on radio advertising from our Chamber of Commerce, I used that to buy a monthly package I otherwise could not have afforded at that time. After my half-price package deal ran its course, a sales representative from the station came around to try to sell me another package. I said to her, "I don't want another ad. I want an interview. How can I get interviewed on your station?" She was taken aback, and said she would have to take that question back to the station manager. He called and said I could have a five-minute interview for $25! I wrote my own script—conveying all the things I wanted the public to know about my business—what we do, who we are, where we're located, the hours we operate, and so forth. As soon as it aired, people started calling me to tell me they had heard me on the radio.

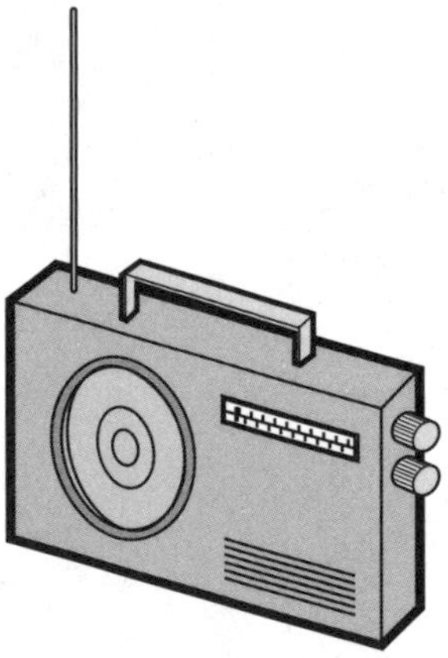

Other Ways to Toot Your Horn Cheaply

Paying for an expensive monthly package year-round is still something I don't want to do, even now. I have cultivated a friendly relationship with the sales managers at a couple of local stations, and I provide them with free gift certificates that they can use for promotional giveaways in exchange for—you've got it—free advertising. On Valentine's Day I give away a free couple's massage that gets mentioned on the air all day until the station does the drawing during afternoon drive time. I have also asked them to notify me whenever they have one-shot deals that I could sponsor at minimal cost, instead of committing myself to a package deal. I have sponsored election results, ACC basketball tournaments, Christmas Eve music, and other one-time events that attract a lot of listeners for much less money than I would spend on an expensive on-going package.

Another good idea is to ask the radio station to keep you informed of events where they will be doing live remotes. Many times, these are outdoor events that attract a lot of passersby, at car dealerships or other businesses. Approach these business owners and ask them if you can do chair massage during their event. Nine times out of ten, they'll be glad to let you participate. Then be sure to give the dee jay (and the business owner who graciously allowed you to participate) a neck and shoulder rub, and ask if he could mention your business as well. You're not trying to take over the event—but they could easily mention you in the context of something like this: "WMMS is broadcasting live out here today in front of Bob's Used Cars, and boy, are we having fun. Bob is giving away free hot dogs and door prizes, and you can get a free chair massage from Melissa of Daylily Day Spa." If you can possibly afford it, a remote broadcast from your business is a great idea. Depending on where you live and the size and market of the station, this might cost you anywhere from a few hundred dollars to a couple of thousand, but in our area they usually attract a lot of people. You might share the cost with a neighboring chiropractor, salon, or other similar business, if there's one nearby, or again, trade part of the cost for free massage and gift certificates. Try offering the station manager the trade of Christmas gift certificates for the station staff. Even if that's a couple of dozen people, you're spending your time instead of laying out cash, and you can spread those redemptions out over the course of the year so they don't wreck your paycheck.

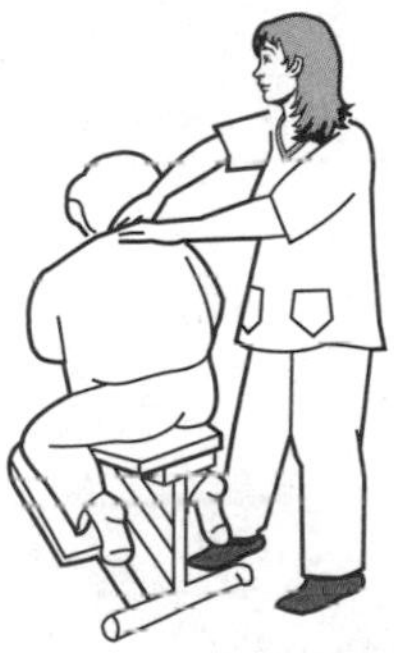

During Massage Therapy Awareness Week, a therapist from my AMTA chapter arranged to go to a local radio station and massage the disc jockeys while they were on the air. For about ten minutes, the public heard the ooohs and aaaahs as the dee jays got their chair massage, during which the name of her business was mentioned several times, followed by a professionally made commercial touting the fact that it was Massage Therapy Awareness Week and urging the public to visit the massage therapist of their choice. It was great and she got a lot of calls from it.

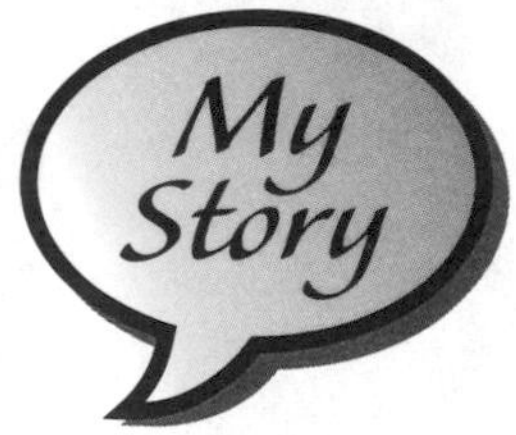

Rachelle's Story

Every year during Massage Therapy Awareness Week (MTWA), I sponsor a whole day of music on one of our local radio stations. I live in a small town and they let me sponsor the whole day for $300, plus the rest of the week, they continue giving public service announcements about MTWA and massage in general. $300 seems like a lot of money, but when you consider that my name is mentioned on the air literally dozens of times on that particular day, it is well worth it. I never book any massage appointments on that day—I'm too busy answering the phone from callers who heard about us on the radio. It's a good value for the money, and I always get at least ten or twelve new appointments out of it, more than enough to cover the cost.

Choosing a Station

Public radio is another possible venue, and should be considered when you are choosing a station to advertise with. The reason for this is just what the name implies: it's public radio, and it's supported by the public. It's on the air because the listeners donate enough funds to keep it going. If someone has enough discretionary money to donate to public radio, they probably have enough to pay for massage. Public radio doesn't accept advertising per se, but they do accept sponsors. If the programming and sponsorship on our local public channel is any indication, a lot of the supporters are holistically minded people. I've gotten my business mentioned for free many times by participating in their annual pledge week. I not only donate a couple of gift certificates for free massage they give to the people who pledge their support, I also take my massage chair and work on the volunteers who are there answering the phones taking pledges. That's usually good for a couple of on-air mentions about how much the phone workers are enjoying their massage, not to mention gathering a couple of new customers. Every time the dee jay mentions the prizes they are giving away, my name is included on the list of donors—and they also thank you with a newspaper ad and an ad in their own newsletter after the event that mentions all the sponsors that participated.

If you live in a small town, you may be limited in your choice of stations. I think it's funny that here in my county, which area-wise is the largest in North Carolina, in addition to our award-winning public radio station, WNCW, there is one country music station, and four stations with religious programming. No rock and roll, no easy listening, no talk radio. The popular stations that play these and other genres are located fifty to one hundred miles or more away, and because of the size of the cities they are located in their market—they're out of my league for advertising. I don't think there's any research proving that people who listen to public radio or rock and roll stations get massage more often than people who listen to country music, so go with the station where you can get the best deal.

When you can't afford expensive advertising, there's always another way to get it. You just have to be a little creative, ask for what you want, and be willing to give away some massage in exchange for it.

My Personal Journey

This Week's Activity: Cheap Advertising on the Radio Date ____________________

For this week's activity, you are going to see if you can get on the radio for free—or for a very minimal cost. Small, local radio stations are usually your best bet. If you live in a big city or metropolitan area, you may have to work a little harder to get some free air time, but it can be done. Call the station manager and offer to come over to massage the disc jockeys and the office staff in exchange for some free radio time. Ask for an on-air interview; keep Massage Therapy Awareness Week in mind (always the first full week in October) as a time when radio stations might be willing to give free public service announcements about massage in general.

My Goals

____

____

____

What's in my way?

____

____

____

What action can I take to remedy the situation?

____

____

____

One-Year Progress Update Date ____________________

____

____

____

POSITIVE AFFIRMATION: **The name of my business is spread far and wide.**

CHAPTER 22

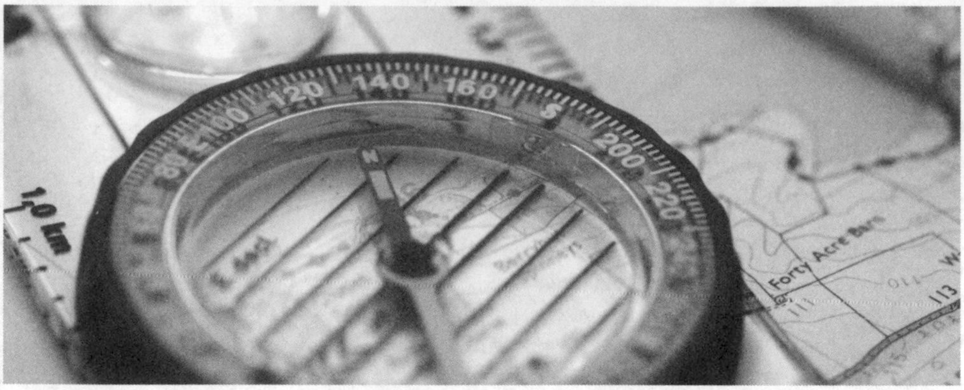

The Awesome Power of the Internet

There are people who make things happen, people who watch what happens, and people who wonder what happened. To be a success, you have to be a person who makes things happen.

—James Lovell

The Internet has made the world a very small place and has changed the face of commerce forever. Even if you're just a one-person operation, don't overlook the value of the Internet in relation to your business.

Spend a Little, Spend a Lot

The Internet can provide your business with many services and advertising opportunities, at any cost from free to as much as you care to spend. The possibilities are endless, but there are also a lot of pitfalls to be avoided. By using the Internet wisely and with caution, you can grow your business, offer conveniences to your customers, and spread information all over the world with the click of a button, at a very reasonable cost.

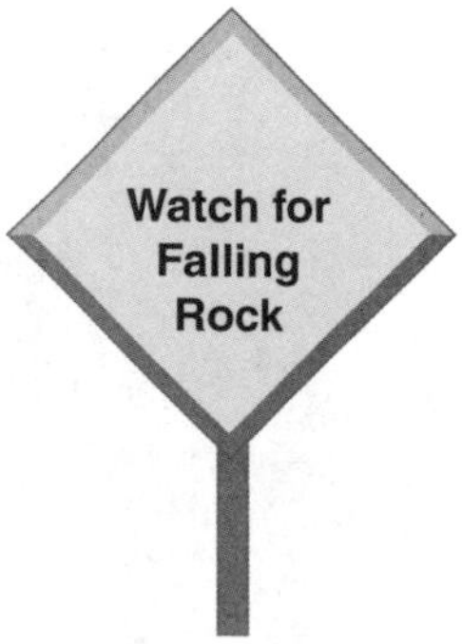

E-mail

By managing your customer information, you can use e-mail for many things. On my intake form, I ask clients for their e-mail address with the specific qualifier, "if you'd like to be notified by e-mail of events or reminded of your appointments." That way, I am not intruding on anyone's privacy; they have asked me to contact them that way. This saves me a lot of money on postage when I'm sending out my quarterly newsletter. I can also send people e-mail reminders of their appointments.

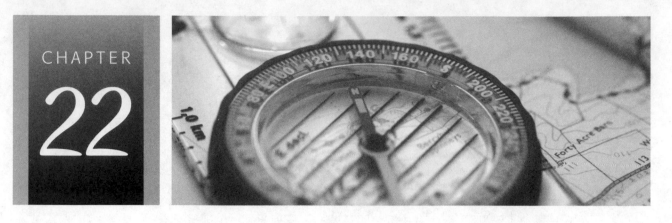

I also keep a separate e-mail folder for people who aren't clients yet; I collect those addresses at health fairs, street festivals, community service events, and so forth, and I also send them copies of the newsletter and announcements about specials and events. Always, I end the e-mail with an opportunity for the recipient to unsubscribe, if they choose. Remember, these people have willingly provided me with their e-mail address.

There are plenty of programs available that allow you to harvest the "cookies," or address, of every person who visits your website, so that you may then spam them with unsolicited messages. Please don't resort to this tactic. If you are respectful of people's privacy, you will do better in the long run.

Your Website

There are a lot of sites on the Web that allow you to build your own free website and will even host your site at no charge. Frankly, forget about them. The downside to them is that your URL, or Internet address, will wind up being something long and obscure, such as www.lauraallenhealingmassageworld@swedishmassageconnection.com. That won't fit on a business card and people can't remember it. Furthermore, some of these companies haven't been in business long enough to have proved they have staying power.

I have a reputable Web host (Yahoo) for which I pay the princely sum of $11.95 per month. My package came with software that is extremely creative and user-friendly to help you build your own website, which can be as simple or as complicated as you want it to be. I chose to use it and built my own, and I enjoy playing around with it and making frequent updates to the site, and have even cultivated a sideline business of building sites for other practitioners; they're nothing fancy, just basic information presented in an attractive way. Since I'm tooting my horn, please visit my site at www.thera-ssage.com.

If you don't feel like that's your forte, somewhere out there is a Web designer just waiting to barter with you for massage. You can spend a fortune on a flashy website, but that's not necessary. People are looking for information, not bells and whistles, unless you're trying to sell your services as a graphic designer.

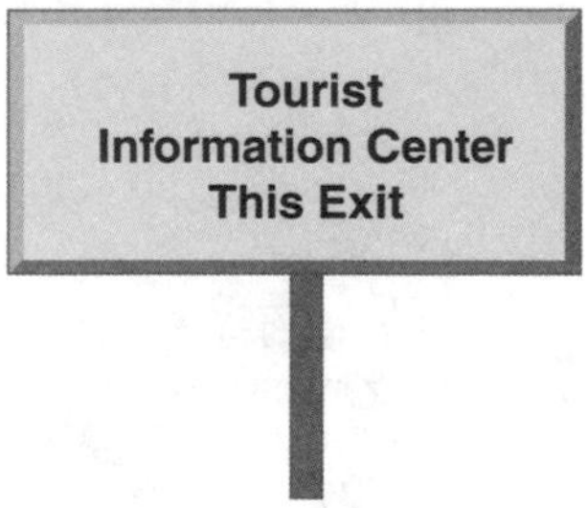

My website has information about the services we offer, special package deals, the educational classes we teach, has bios of all of our staff members, archives of past newsletters, and more. It gets more hits with each passing month, and even though I have never paid for any type of search engine placement, it is at the top of the search engine list for massage therapists in my area. The Web address is on our business cards and all other literature. Any time someone calls to find out what type of services we offer, I always ask them if they have Internet access, and give them the Web address if they do. That frees up my time, and gives the customer something nice to look at with much more detail than I have time to give them on the phone.

You can also sell gift certificates or retail items from your website; have an e-mail form to make it easy for people to e-mail you with questions or to sign up for your free newsletter, and so forth. There are even Web services that allow you to display your schedule and let clients book appointments right over the Internet. A website doesn't have to cost much and it can really pay off for your business.

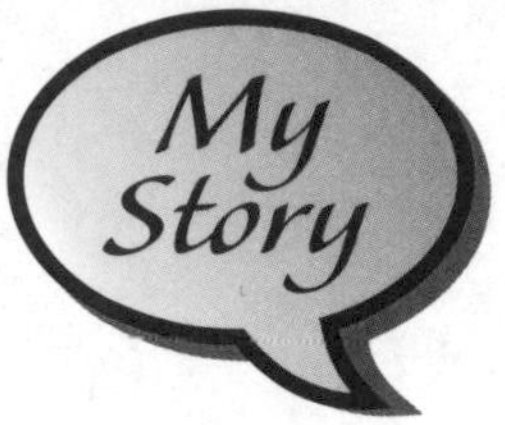

Queenie's Story

My gift certificate sales have increased dramatically since I got a website and made it possible for people to order them on-line. They have the option of my mailing the certificate to their recipient, or they can actually print out a certificate on their end if they prefer. Having a website is a general enhancement to my business, but this has been the most tangible result.

Listing Services

It seems like every day I get a solicitation from a new Internet massage listing service. Some of these are free; if that's the case, you should definitely take advantage of it, because every little bit helps. If it's a paid service, examine the fine print carefully. There is a lot of variance in the price of these paid services. I belong to a few that I am paying $50–100 per year to be listed on. I have turned down a lot of others that wanted $300 or more to have a listing on their site. Unless you have an unlimited budget, choose carefully those Internet services you pay for. One that I am listed on is www.massageresource.com That's a straightforward name, and comes out near the top of search engine queries, so it's a good value. Avoid paid listing services that have obscure names and Internet addresses. They're not worth the money.

If you belong to a professional association, chances are you can be listed on their practitioner pages for free. The Massage Locator service on the website of the American Massage Therapy Association is getting hundreds of thousands of hits per month.

Others that are reputable and have staying power, such as the National Certification Board for Therapeutic Massage & Bodywork and Associated Bodywork & Massage Professionals, are listed in Appendices II and IV.

Reciprocal Links

You can get a lot of free Internet exposure by exchanging links with other sites. *Be extremely careful about this.* Any time you place your link, carefully peruse the entire site that you are thinking of linking to, and make sure that not only is there no adult content, gambling solicitations, or any other questionable things you don't want massage associated with on the site, but also that there are no links to such sites on that site. It may be time-consuming to go carefully through every page of a big website, but don't link to one until you've done just that.

My own website has a link page that contains links to massage schools, supply vendors that I use, other teachers I admire, other practitioners in other towns that I refer to, professional associations, and so forth. I also have a link inviting others to send a link, and I have had to turn many of them down for just those reasons. Maybe their actual website didn't contain any porn or gambling, but they had a link *somewhere* on the site that was objectionable. You don't want to be associated with anything like that. Otherwise, some pervert could punch in "massage" and "sex" on the search engine and your website might come up. Peruse every page of any website you are thinking of trading links with very carefully so you won't be at risk for associating yourself with something you don't want to be associated with.

My Personal Journey

This Week's Activity: Utilizing the Internet

Date ______________________

For this week's activity, you are going to start perusing the Internet and developing a plan for Internet marketing. If you don't already have a website, start writing the text to describe your business, your services, and the other information you would include on a website. Gather photographs, either personal and/or stock photos that will complement your text. Write down specifics, such as what colors you'd like to use, how many different pages you would like to include on the site, and so forth. You will not want to put the actual site on the Web until you are licensed (if that's a requirement in your state).

Also work on organizing e-mail addresses so you can use them effectively for client communication.

My Goals

____

____

____

What's in my way?

____

____

____

What action can I take to remedy the situation?

____

____

____

One-Year Progress Update

Date ______________________

____

____

____

POSITIVE AFFIRMATION: **My business can reach the whole world.**

CHAPTER 23

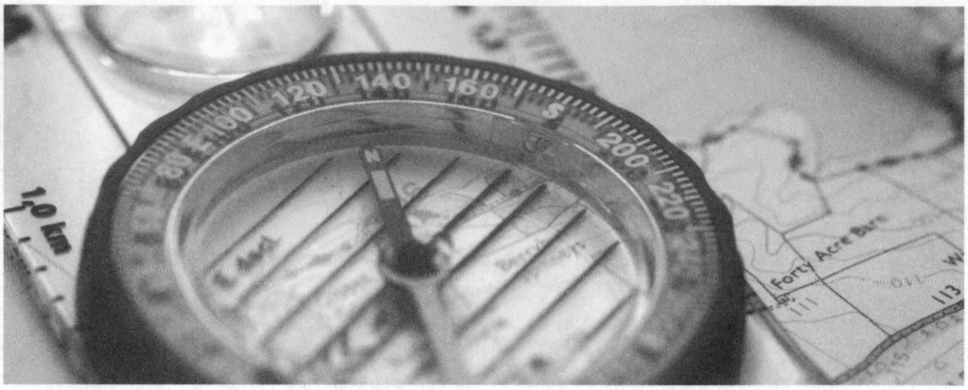

Rescheduling Clients

The elevator to success is out of order. You'll have to use the stairs . . . one step at a time.

—Joe Girard

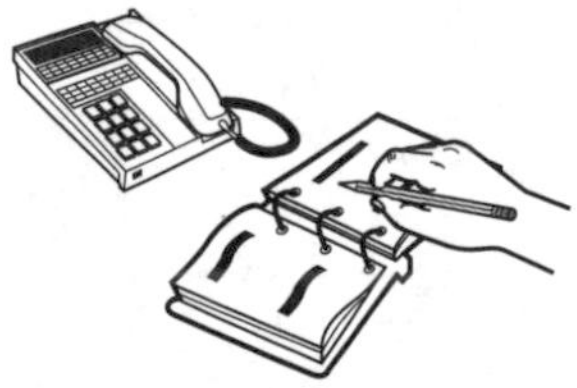

Next to "Thank you," the most important phrase you can offer to clients after their massage is "Would you like to schedule another appointment?"

Unless you are observing silence during the massage as we all do at times, there may be occasion during the actual treatment to bring up the need for more work, or you can broach the subject after the massage as they are preparing to leave; sometimes clients do tell you that they don't want any conversation. You should of course check in with them on the pressure at the beginning and periodically. If someone is in particularly bad condition, such as chronic shoulder or back problems that they have lived with for a long time, gently mention to them during the intake interview that they did not get in this condition overnight, and that one massage, while it is sure to effect some relief, is not going to make it go away. Suggest *before* they even get on the table that you estimate that it would take *x* number of sessions to bring them maximum relief, and that once they are out of pain, they will need to schedule regular maintenance appointments.

If your practice focuses mainly on relaxation therapy, suggest that a massage once a week, once a month, or however often your client can afford it is going to keep them more flexible and less stressed, increase their circulation, and so forth. You can and should let them know the benefits of receiving regular massage, especially if they're new to massage.

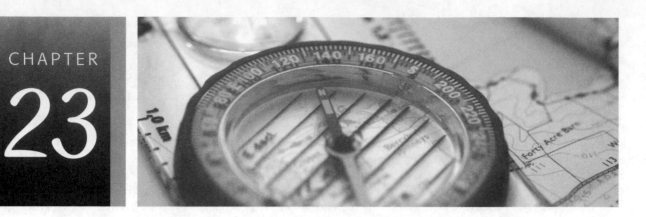

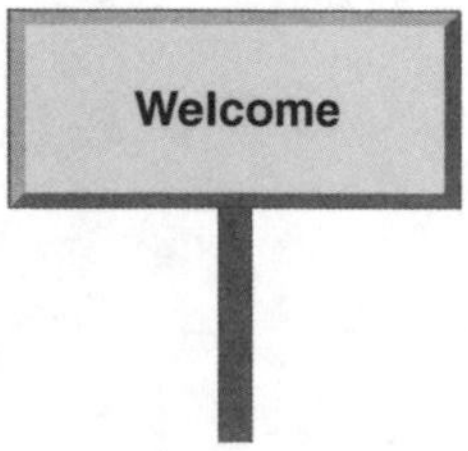

It can make a big difference to your practice if you will follow up with clients, particularly new ones. When a new client comes in, wait a couple of days after their appointment and then give them a call to ask how they have felt since receiving their massage. Send a "welcome to our practice" postcard, and—*if* they didn't book another appointment before leaving—you might want to include a $5 off coupon for their second visit. People have a choice in where to go. Make them aware that you are grateful that they chose your business.

If you don't have a clear picture of how many of your clients fail to reschedule, look at your client files. Say you have 100 files. If 30 of those people have only visited once, then 70% of your customers are repeaters—and you want the others to be repeaters also. Consider sending people you haven't seen in a long time a postcard with a discount coupon on it, or an offer of the free paraffin hand treatment with the purchase of a massage. Mine say, "We haven't seen you in a long time and we'd like to, so here's $5 off on your next massage." It gets people back in. Of course, you may have tourists and out-of-town visitors coming through your business that are just one-timers, and you're not going to pursue them, but if they live in town, go after them!

Evangeline's Story

I was very timid about asking people to reschedule at first, but I forced myself to do it and it has really paid off. The first week I was open for business, I only had five clients, but all five of them rescheduled and are still customers two years later. It's second nature to me now to ask.

Client Incentives

An incentive is something that gives you a reason to take a particular action. In this case, what you want is something that will bring your clients back again—and again. In my office, we use a "buy ten, get one free" deal as a customer reward. Once a client has paid for ten massages (they don't have to pay all at once; that's a different deal that will be discussed in the next section), they receive a gift certificate for a free massage. They're free to use it themselves or to pass it on to someone.

For the once-a-month client, this assures them that once a year, they'll get a free massage. For the client who comes every week or more, it can add up to a substantial reward in a year's time—up to five free massages a year or even more, depending on how often they schedule. You may choose to do yours differently—one free for every twelve or whatever you decide, but the point is to build customer loyalty. Even though I have publicized this deal in our newsletter many times, some clients forget about it, and when they receive their gift certificate, which says "Customer Appreciation," they are just thrilled to get it.

Another incentive may be a reward for client referrals. A therapist I know gives a $5 credit for each referral she receives from an existing client. Before you offer such a deal, make sure it does not conflict with any of the rules governing massage therapy in your particular state or locale. The board rules in some states prohibit giving any gifts to influence a referral.

Package Deals

The "buy ten, get one free" incentive mentioned above is a reward for customer loyalty. So are package deals, special offers you can make to people who can afford to pay up front. I use "buy five, get six" and "buy ten, get twelve" packages. Package sales can help your cash flow a great deal. They can also put you in a financial bind if you aren't careful, especially around holidays when you sell a lot of certificates. You have to remember that the money for those packages is basically in escrow. You've got the money, but you still owe the services. You may have to exercise a little caution when scheduling people. If your goal is 20 clients a week and they've all previously paid for a package deal, you'd be working hard for a week and not getting any cash—you've already received it. Bear that in mind and don't spend all that money at once.

Package deals are an excellent way to get people to commit to regular massage. It cuts their price per massage; it also cuts your profit per massage, but it guarantees a certain amount of repeat business.

You may want to consider making package deals for people who get more than one service in a day. We offer spa services, so for instance if someone books a hot stone massage and a mud wrap on the same day, I'll cut $5 or $10 off just to be nice. I also give discounts to bridal parties or other groups who want to bring several people at the same time, maybe 10% off if at least four people are coming together.

Other therapists have told me that they have great success with their package deals; that it encourages clients to return more often because they're getting the massage at a cheaper rate, and that they have also seen an increase in tips for the same reason. Many of the clients in my office include the tip for the whole package at the time of purchase. For those therapists who have clients who insist on seeing only their favorite therapist, that can mean a $50 or $100 tip on the spot.

To those who are wondering, and to those who may be in the same position I am in—that of having other therapists working as independent contractors in your office—I do not expect therapists to do a "free" massage when a client purchases a package. On the average package deal, the client is paying $10 less per massage. I give up $5, and the therapist gives up $5. In exchange for that sacrifice, we both have the guarantee that the client is going to return at least six times. Most of the time the person purchasing a package will make a standing appointment and book the whole six or twelve right at the time they purchase the package. Any therapist working in my business has the option of not taking clients who are on package deals, and that is made plain to them. In fact, a long-standing therapist did refuse for quite some time to do package massage, but when she realized the repeat business that was coming in on account of package sales, she changed her mind. I do not sell packages on the services of the specialty practitioners who travel to my office to work once a week or so; I just explain to clients that they are traveling too far for me to discount their services, and no one has ever gotten upset about it.

Retrieving Lost Clients

Have you ever wondered what has happened to your clients who have disappeared? Of course you have. But whether or not you have contacted those clients to find out why they've fallen by the wayside may be a different story.

Sometimes therapists feel shy about contacting someone to find out why they're no longer coming for massage. Get over it! Send an e-mail, send a card, send a letter, *but do something*. If the person was a regular client and suddenly stops coming, I am certainly going to call to inquire about their health. You don't have to sound pushy. Here's a script: "Mrs. Lindsay, this is Laura Allen, the massage therapist. It's been two months since I've heard from you and I just wanted to make sure you're doing okay."

Like any other service-oriented business, clients come and go. They die. They move away. Or they get another therapist! Maybe someone opened a massage therapy business very close to their home and they no longer need to drive across town to see you, but you won't know if you don't ask. Here's an exact copy of an e-mail I sent to a client (name changed, of course) who lives about twenty miles away from my office:

> Dear Carmen,
> I haven't seen you in a while. Are you doing okay? I know it's quite a distance for you to come here—if you've gotten another massage therapist closer to home I certainly understand. I just wanted to make sure you're all right. Let me hear from you when you have the time.
> Laura Allen

That's not being pushy; it's being concerned. She immediately responded to me that her absence was due to a serious family matter that resulted in her having to take temporary custody of three young grandchildren—and hence didn't have a free minute to come and get a massage. She assured me she would be back when the situation was resolved, and she has been, but if I hadn't sent the e-mail, I'd still be wondering.

A little healthy introspection may be in order before contacting someone, and maybe a look at their file. How often they were coming and what kind of progress they were making could be a big factor for them, if for instance it was a rehabilitative injury client. They may have had different expectations for the length and outcome of their treatment than you did, particularly if you did not discuss that at length with them.

If you're courteous, professional, and on time for *every client*, your office is clean beyond reproach, you act ethically and you take time to listen to people, you can assume you are not at fault in any meaningful way. You can't take it personally every time someone doesn't come back, but that doesn't mean you shouldn't try to find out if there's a problem. Sometimes the reason is money; sometimes it's something like they've changed shifts at work and can no longer come during your operating hours. Once per quarter, I look through my records for people who haven't been in the past three months and send them the previously mentioned postcard. We get a lot of people back that way. Of course, if the client was someone who was a frequent visitor who suddenly disappeared, I will make the call long before three months have passed, maybe a month at the most. Some therapists may feel it's too invasive to call at all. If that applies to you, stick to sending a postcard or a personal letter. At least you will know you have made an effort to get the client back.

My Personal Journey

This Week's Activity: Rescheduling Clients Date ____________________

For this week's activity, you are going to start tracking the number of clients who rebook, and take action to increase that number. Let's work on percentages. If you have twenty clients in a week, and six of them rebook, that's a little more than 33%. What can you do to bump that up to at least 50%, and on a consistent basis? Formulate your plan for client incentives, customer rewards, package deals, and so forth. Also, get in the habit of asking every single client to rebook. A simple method of keeping track is to put a checkmark by their name when they agree to rebook (in addition, of course, to putting the appointment on the calendar). That way, you can quickly look back, count the total number of clients you had, and use the checkmarks to figure the percentage who rebooked.

My Goals

____

____

____

What's in my way?

____

____

____

What action can I take to remedy the situation?

____

____

____

One-Year Progress Update Date ____________________

____

____

____

POSITIVE AFFIRMATION: **My clients look forward to returning to my business.**

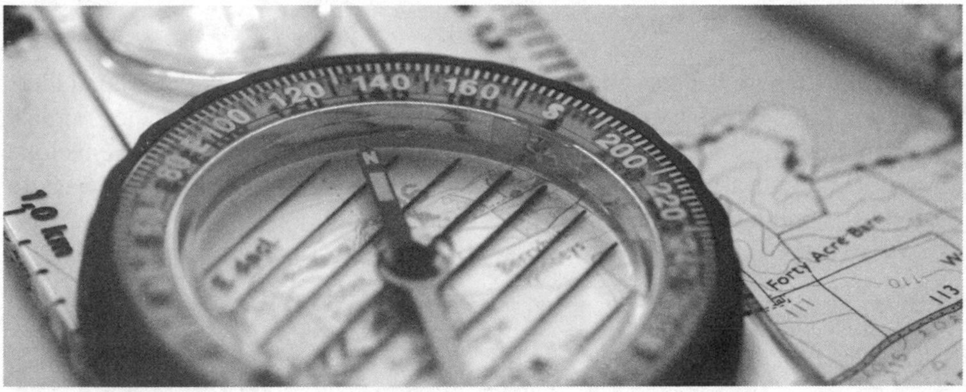

CHAPTER

24

Take a Survey

A minute's success pays the failure of years.

—Robert Browning

Marketing consultants have always relied on surveys to find out what the public wants. Since the exponential growth of the Internet, the opinions of thousands of people can be harvested in minutes.

Taking a survey can give you the facts about what the consumers in your area want—and/or what the clients you already have would like to see changed or added to your business. You can send them by e-mail, direct mail, or hand them to clients when they come in the door and ask them to fill them out. The response rate on surveys is typically low—if 3% of direct mail gets a response that's considered a success—so don't get discouraged. The theory is that a small sample represents the majority of the whole.

Your survey could look like this:

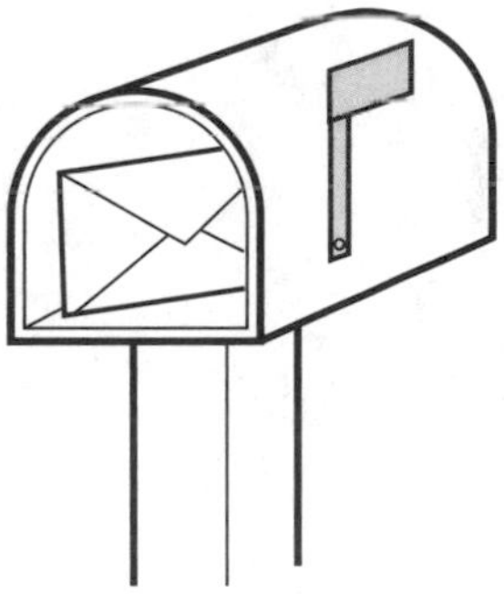

The Body Shop Survey

Dear Customer,

Please help us in our quest to serve you better by answering the following questions:

Are our days and hours of operation convenient for you? yes ❑ no ❑

If not, what days/hours would you like to see us extend? ____________________

Do you think our prices are too high ❑ too low ❑ reasonable ❑

Are there other services that you wish we would offer? ____________________

Do you find our facility to be clean and comfortable? yes ❑ no ❑

Have you ever referred anyone to us for massage? yes ❑ no ❑

Is there anything else we could do to improve your experience? yes ❑ no ❑

If so, please tell us what we could do to serve you better: ____________________

You may have other questions that you want to ask, but you get the general idea. People tend to be more honest when surveys are anonymous. You can accomplish this by mailing the surveys to your clients—enclose postcard surveys in an envelope for mailing, and instruct them that it is an anonymous survey and to mail it back to you without putting their name on it.

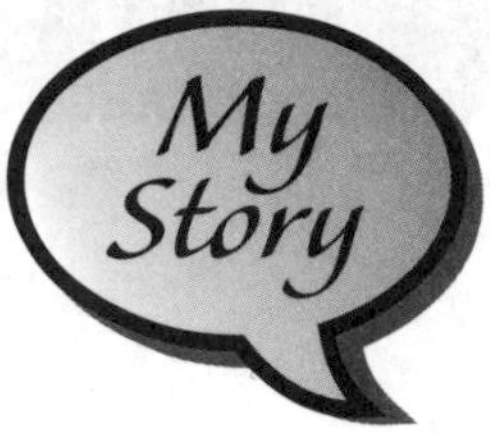

Gabby's Story

I took a survey of my clients, and found that what they wanted more than anything was for me to start accepting credit cards. That wasn't a priority for me when I opened my business, but after I saw how many people requested it on the survey, I decided I needed to offer that service.

If you should decide to do a bulk direct mail survey to a broader audience, say everyone in your zip code, you'll want to add a few questions at the beginning, such as "Have you ever visited The Body Shop?" "Why not?" and so forth. That's a much more expensive undertaking, one that I wouldn't do unless I was also going to include a coupon for first-time clients on it. That way, you would at least stand a chance of getting new business along with spending your money on the survey. You could also try sending these out to those clients who have fallen by the wayside, as a method of finding out why they are no longer patronizing your business.

My Personal Journey

This Week's Activity: Taking a Survey Date ____________________

For this week's activity, you are going to take a survey. If you're still a student, you can adapt this survey by asking questions such as "If I open my own massage office, what hours would you like me to keep?" and so forth. If you're an existing practitioner, this may give you some insight into what you could be doing better or differently. The purpose of any survey is market research—what does the target market want, how often or how much do they want it, how much are they willing to pay for it, and other similar questions. Of course, everyone you survey may want something different (depending on how small or large a group you survey), but chances are you'll find *something* that a number of people have in common, and usually what the majority asks for are good things to implement.

My Goals

____

____

____

What's in my way?

____

____

____

What action can I take to remedy the situation?

____

____

____

One-Year Progress Update Date ____________________

____

____

____

POSITIVE AFFIRMATION: **My advertisements attract attention wherever they are.**

CHAPTER

25

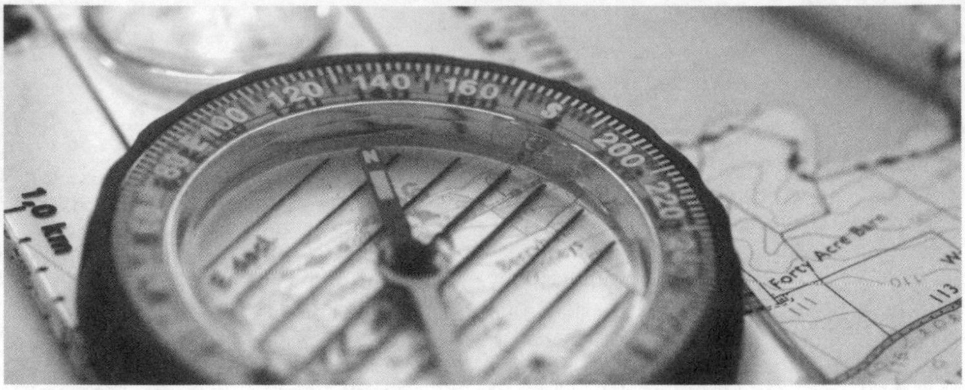

Two-fers

Whenever I hear "It can't be done," I know I'm close to success.

—MICHAEL FLATLEY

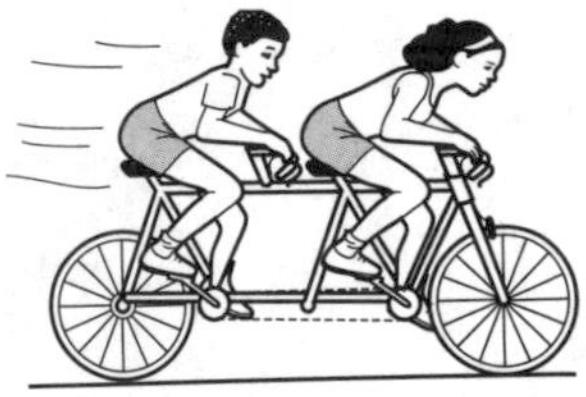

Two-fers is just a fun term for *two for the price of one*. Why would you even consider giving two massages for the price of one? Because, one of those people is going to be someone you've never met before—a potential new client.

Make the offer to all of your existing clients that you will give them a "two-fer," so they can bring a friend or family member. You have to put some stipulations on it in order for it to have the desired effect:

1. It has to be someone who has never been to your business before, and
2. It has to be someone who lives in your town (or whatever radius you feel comfortable with)—the point is, you don't want to make that offer to the relative from Alaska who's never coming back. If there's no potential for you to get a new client, it's a fruitless exercise.

If you work alone and can't take two people at once (you can always schedule one after the other), a further good stipulation might be that they come if not on the same day, at least during the same week or month. You don't want the deal to drag on. You may also want to make it good for half-hour massages instead of an hour, with the option to upgrade to a longer session at a higher price; or go to the other extreme and make it something special like "hot stone" massage or some other modality you'd like to increase the sales of. If you do have staff members, it will be up to you to make a fair arrangement with them regarding the pay for this service. Getting new business will serve both of you in the long run, but you can't expect your therapists to do two for the price of one and still take your usual cut, assuming you want to keep a happy staff. Sit down with them and work it out.

Put a short expiration date on the offer when you make it, and do it during what is a slow time for you. You don't want to be stressing out over fitting people in during the holidays—do your "two-fer" during September, January, or whatever is a slow time for you. Of course, if you're just starting out in business, any time is a good time.

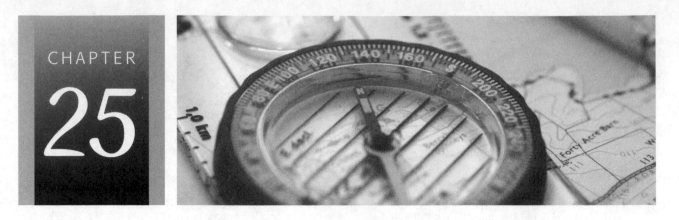

Fontaine's Story

I offered "two-fers" the whole first month I was in business, and the results were great; I got my practice off to a good start. I still occasionally do it during the slower winter months, and it always brings in some new customers. I also just offer it to some of my regular clients, if they say something like, "I've been trying to get my daughter (or whomever) in here for a massage." It rewards the regular client with a cheaper massage and brings in new people, too.

My Story

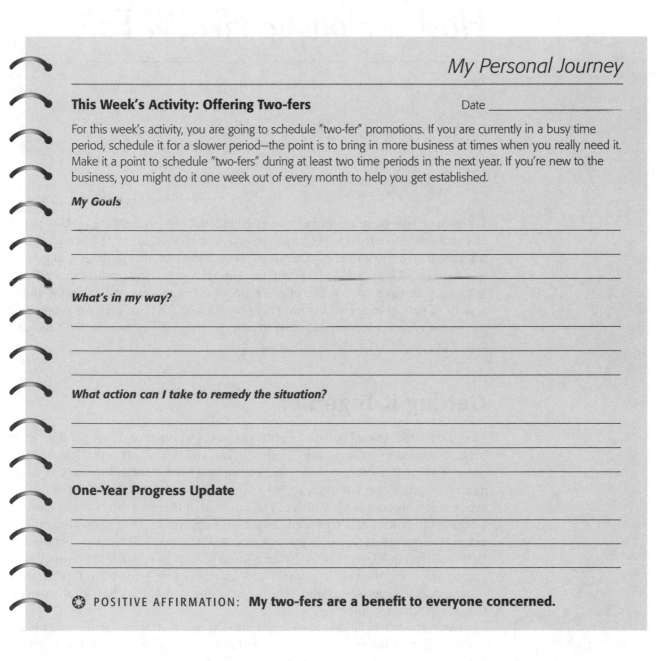

My Personal Journey

This Week's Activity: Offering Two-fers Date ____________________

For this week's activity, you are going to schedule "two-fer" promotions. If you are currently in a busy time period, schedule it for a slower period—the point is to bring in more business at times when you really need it. Make it a point to schedule "two-fers" during at least two time periods in the next year. If you're new to the business, you might do it one week out of every month to help you get established.

My Goals

What's in my way?

What action can I take to remedy the situation?

One-Year Progress Update

POSITIVE AFFIRMATION: **My two-fers are a benefit to everyone concerned.**

CHAPTER

26

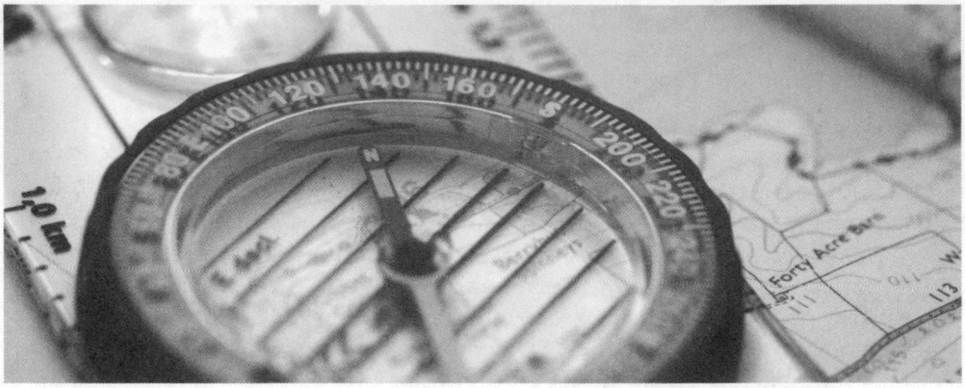

Host a Holistic Health Fair

Success is liking yourself, liking what you do, and liking how you do it.
—Maya Angelou

Hosting a holistic health fair can be a big undertaking—depending on how grand an event you'd like for it to be. It can be done on a small scale, with just a few practitioners in your own office space, or it can be a big deal that requires you getting a space to hold it in. A holistic health fair can serve a lot of purposes: to publicize not only your business, but that of other practitioners as well, which has the added benefit of getting to network with other practitioners; to raise cash for yourself or for a charity; and most importantly, to educate the public that you don't have to take a pill for everything that ails you.

Getting It Together

I have attended several holistic health fairs in larger cities and thought they were great. I wanted to so something similar in my small town. It was a lot of work, but it was such a success and a marketing bonanza, I intend to have it as an annual event. Since I wanted to have something on a grand scale, I needed a space much bigger than my office. The purpose of this was not to make money; I decided to hold it as a charitable event, so I approached the town council and asked for free use of the town gymnasium. Ask and ye shall receive. I chose the first weekend in November as the date—and used it to kick off the holiday season by requiring the public to make a donation of non-perishable food or new unwrapped toys as admission. These were donated to the Salvation Army's Christmas Cheer Center.

Once you have chosen a date and secured a place, start contacting other practitioners. I used my own contact list, and asked their help in contacting others. Here's a sample letter you can send out:

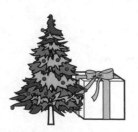

THERA-SSAGE
431 S. Main St., Ste. 2
Rutherfordton NC 28139

Dear Fellow Practitioner of the Healing Arts,

THERA-SSAGE is going to host a Holistic Health Fair at the Cool Springs Gymnasium on Saturday, November 1, from 9am-1pm. We would love for you to participate. The cost of a 10′ × 10′ booth space is only $50 and includes an 8-foot table and two chairs for your use. You must supply your own table coverings. Electrical outlets are limited and vendors who need electricity will be accommodated on a first-come, first-served basis.

Please contact me immediately at 828-288-3727 if you are interested in participating. This event will be heavily advertised, and will give us all the opportunity to introduce the public to what we do. We hope you will be able to join us for this great day of wellness and education.

Peace and Prosperity,

Laura Allen, LMBT

I used the Internet to search for holistic practitioners, and obtained copies of regional health and holistic magazines that practitioners advertise in as another source. Out of 150 letters I mailed out asking for participants, I got 45 practitioners to pay for a booth space. That money was used to advertise the event, and to buy a huge banner that hung in front of the gym for six weeks before the event. Since it was for charity, I got quite a bit of free advertising as well in the form of public service announcements. I sent press releases to every radio and television station within a 100-mile radius.

I also put a page on my website about the fair, and as a result, practitioners called me from two other states and from a town on the coast more than eight hours away, and rented booths—it had never occurred to me that people would travel so far!

NEWS FLASH!

Benefits Galore

I was overwhelmed at the response. There were chiropractors, acupuncturists, people doing aura readings, energy workers, aromatherapy, people who made natural products such as organic soaps and hemp clothing. There were also naturopaths, homeopaths, herbalists; it was really incredible. I also invited every massage therapist in our county; three different massage schools participated. There was no competition. The chiropractors all visited each other's stations, the massage therapists and students were giving each other massage during slow periods—and there weren't many—and it was just a beautiful spirit of wellness and community. I gave a health food store owner a free booth who agreed to provide organic food, juices, and bottled water so there would be food available at the event.

I had expected, erroneously, that the majority of attendees would be the younger, hip set. I was gratified and amazed at the number of senior citizens who attended. A lady who was in her late 80s lay right down on a pad on the floor for a Shiatsu session. Seniors were lined up at the Chi machine, the reflexology station, and the aura readings. We collected a lot of food and toys, everyone had a great time, everyone learned something new, and it was just a fabulous event.

The amount of publicity that I got from the event was such that six months later, practitioners from all over are already calling wanting to know when we're doing another one. The local shopper paper, which is distributed for free to thousands of people, had it on the front page—no charge; it was advertised on the TV guide of the cable company—no charge; the banner, which was seen for six weeks by everyone on Main Street and the ads that were paid were paid for by the booth rental—no cost out of my pocket; it was announced on numerous radio stations—no charge, and every single ad and announcement said "Sponsored by THERASSAGE" (the name of my business)—no charge. In addition, I asked every practitioner who participated to post it on their websites—probably 30 out of the 45 participants have one—again, no charge. And don't forget—whatever advertising you do pay for, and any other expenses incurred as a result of this fair and your other promotional activities are tax-deductible. Keep careful track of your expenses on the first go-round, and you'll have a base figure to work with the next time you plan an event like this.

On top of the free advertising, my business probably gained about a dozen new clients as a result of the event. While I invested probably 30–40 hours of time over a two-month period in organizing the event, the return that I have received has been magnanimous. The public service announcements alone would have cost me thousands of dollars. All in all, it was one of the most successful events I have ever participated in. The publicity and good will it generated were priceless.

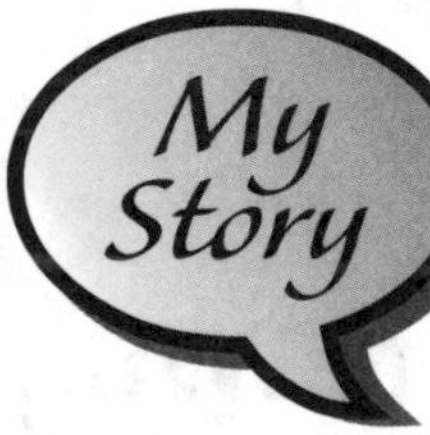

Richard's Story

I share an office with an acupuncturist and an energy worker. We've all participated in other health fairs, so we decided to hold one of our own. We're located next door to a private school and we were able to rent their gym at a reasonable price, to have it in. We had twenty exhibitors, including a chiropractor, a midwife, a colon hydrotherapist, and other alternative health practitioners. We weren't in it for the money, just the publicity. We had a good turnout and felt like we really introduced people to some things they might not have been aware of. The school held a bake sale and a car wash in front of the gym on the same day, so we mutually helped each other's attendance. It was a big success.

"Nitty-Gritty" Details

Whenever you arrange for your venue to hold the fair in, you want to be sure you have all the pertinent details and are well prepared. The manager should be able to tell you the square footage of the room. If they can't, whip out your tape measure. You need to know how much space you have so you will know how many vendors you can accept. I rented the booth spaces as 10' × 10' spaces, and of course, people were free to rent more than one if they needed extra space. While you're measuring, you will also need to count how many electric outlets are available. I invested quite a bit of money in power strips with surge protection and extension cords. You can require people to bring those, but I think things ran more smoothly in the setup and breakdown, because I already had those plugged in and taped down with duct tape so there wouldn't be any tripping over cords.

Find out if tables and chairs come with the building. If not, require everyone to bring their own. That should be detailed in the letter you send inviting them to participate, along with any other requirements you care to have. Some festivals are very insistent that people use only 6-foot banquet tables, no card tables, have their tables draped and skirted, or require everyone to have the same color tablecloths so it will look nice. If that's important to you, detail that in the letter as well, when you let the vendors know your expectations for the event. Also let the vendors know if they need to provide a trash can and/or bags for themselves.

I also had a person at the door collecting the food and toys (or a donation if the attendee failed to bring something), and another person patrolling between the parking lot and entrance to assist elderly and handicapped people with parking and getting in. Since we were given free use of the building, we also had to agree to clean it up afterwards.

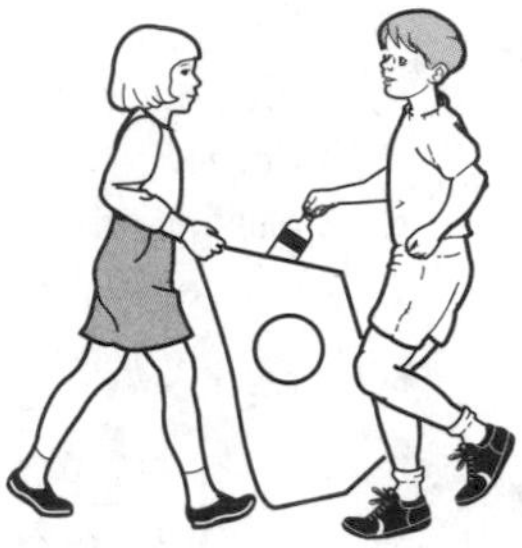

Same Idea, Smaller Scale

If you don't feel ready to do something on as big a scale, invite two or three other practitioners of different healing arts, or as many as will comfortably fit in your office. Or get ten and hold it in your church Fellowship Hall. The concept is the same though the logistics may differ.

The public service announcement could read:

> The Massage Room will be hosting a Holistic Health Fair on Saturday, May 20, at their office on Maple Street. Dana Goforth, Doctor of Naturopathy, Dr. Denny Seal, chiropractor, and Jeff Wilson, acupuncturist, will be doing consultations in exchange for at least $10 worth of nonperishable food items that will be donated to the Grace Homeless Shelter. Call 288-8888 for more information.

Whether your fair is big or small, you're still bringing in people who will benefit from learning something new, meeting potential new clients, sharing opportunities with other practitioners, and supporting a worthwhile cause in one clip. It's a "win-win" situation.

My Personal Journey

This Week's Activity: Organizing a Holistic Health Fair Date ______________________

For this week's activity, you are going to plan a Holistic Health Fair. If you're still a student, this would make a great graduation project for you. If they have the space, the massage school might even be a great place to hold it. Talk with your director if that seems like a feasible idea. If you're in practice, locate a venue (even your own office, if you have enough room for other participants and the public to come in) and choose a date. Compose a letter about your proposed health fair and send it out to as many practitioners and vendors as you will have room for (and more—not everyone will be able to participate). Send out press announcements about your event.

My Goals

____

____

____

What's in my way?

____

____

____

What action can I take to remedy the situation?

____

____

____

One-Year Progress Update

____

____

____

POSITIVE AFFIRMATION: **Educating the public is fun and profitable.**

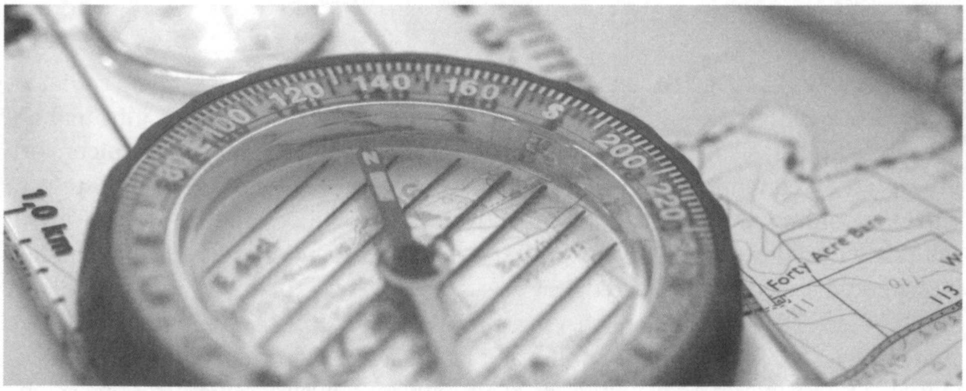

CHAPTER 27

Have a Mentor, Be a Mentor

Success is a consequence and must not be a goal.

—GUSTAVE FLAUBERT

A mentor is someone to look up to, to turn to for advice, whose experience and expertise exceed yours, and whose opinion you value and trust. At any given time, I am mentoring three or four students. At any given time, I have at least two or three mentors of my own.

One of my mentors is a sharp lady that I took a marketing class from a few years ago. Although I was already teaching marketing myself at the time, I still like to go to other people's classes for fresh ideas. Felicia graduated from massage school, got an office and another therapist to share a room in it. Eight years later, she had a facility that had fifteen treatment rooms, more than eighty employees, and her bottom line was several million dollars a year when she decided to sell the business and devote her self to teaching and consulting full time. That's the kind of person I want rooting for me and helping me along.

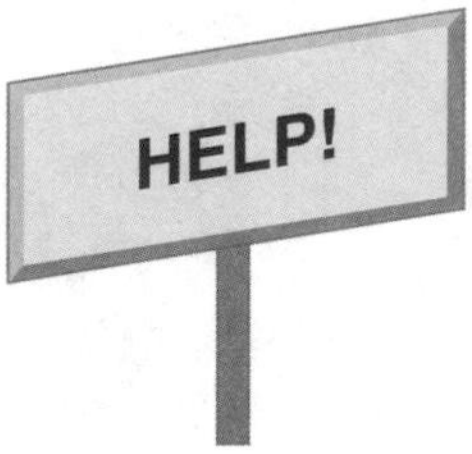

Another mentor is a former teacher of mine from massage school who has had a steady twenty-five clients a week for the past ten years. Instead of a multi-million dollar facility, she practices out of a trailer that she has turned into her office, in a very small rural community. She attracts clients like flies to honey, because she's an effective therapist and her clients are constantly sending her referrals.

Mentors aren't afraid of competition. They welcome it. They believe there are enough aching bodies to go around—and they're right. If you open yourself to advice, there are plenty of therapists who share that philosophy, and who will be willing to help you on your way. Sometimes a mentor may tell you something you don't want to hear—and that's the very thing you need to listen to. A mentor may share marketing ideas, or they may tell you that when they got a massage from you, they couldn't help but notice all the dust bunnies under the massage table. A mentor can be a friend or a colleague; a coach to help you attain success. A mentor is someone to talk to when faced with a problem you need a fresh perspective on.

If you think you don't need a mentor, reconsider that attitude. By the nature of what we do, placing our hands on unclothed people, and being bound to observe confidentiality, we do face ethical dilemmas and difficult situations from time to time. There will be times when you need moral support. Sometimes, in the advancement of our careers, or in the spirit of community service, we take on jobs that are stressful and that seem overwhelming; for instance, volunteering for hospice work or serving on committees and boards. I recall a student who worked in a hospice to meet her community service requirement for massage school, telling me how awful she felt when she showed up week after week, and found that the people she had massaged the week before had died.

As I am writing this, I am serving a term on our state massage board. We are charged with safeguarding the public, and I have to participate in disciplinary hearings of therapists who have been charged with unethical conduct. It's one of the most stressful things I have ever done—to have to decide whether someone is innocent or guilty and perhaps take away their license and their livelihood. I leave every meeting wondering if I did the right thing. It's particularly difficult when board members disagree and I'm in the minority. If I didn't have a mentor to talk to about that, I'd probably be taking anti-anxiety drugs, or having an emotional meltdown on the way home.

While a mentor can certainly be a friend, that's not a requirement. Sometimes, it might be better if they're not. A mentor needs to be brutally honest at times, and you might hold it against a friend if they told you your office was looking dirty or that you need to quit taking those garlic pills that are making you stink!

If you don't have anyone in particular in mind to be your mentor, you might consider calling your local chapter of SCORE, the Service Corps of Retired Executives. These are retired business people from all walks of life, who volunteer their time to give help and business advice to entrepreneurs who need it. One of the benefits of belonging to the Chamber of Commerce in our town is a free matching service to a SCORE mentor. Our Chamber will find a mentor who has expertise in your particular area—financial advice, ethics, or whatever you require.

If you're fresh out of school, it isn't time for you to be a mentor, yet. After you've got a few years of experience under your belt, I hope you'll be a mentor for others who need the benefit of your experience. Helping people never hurt anyone—just the opposite. It's a great honor to be asked to mentor someone, and an opportunity to serve our profession.

My Story

Mary's Story

My mentor jokes with me that my name is really "Mary-just-one-more-question," but it's been really important to me my first couple of years in the business to have someone that's more experienced I can call on. Sometimes it's advice, sometimes just a pep talk; either way, it's great to be able to turn to someone who's been through the same things I have and survived and prospered. As I gain more experience and self-confidence, I plan to do the same for someone else.

My Personal Journey

This Week's Activity: Getting a Mentor/Being a Mentor Date ____________

This week's activity, if you are still a student or new practitioner, is to contact at least two experienced therapists and ask them to mentor you. If you are an experienced practitioner, offer to mentor a new therapist just starting out. And even if you are experienced, you should still have someone to mentor you—someone you can turn to for a fresh perspective. Make the necessary contacts, whether you are giving or receiving (and as you'll discover as time goes by, that's the same thing).

My Goals

____

____

____

What's in my way?

____

____

____

What action can I take to remedy the situation?

____

____

____

One-Year Progress Update Date ____________

____

____

____

POSITIVE AFFIRMATION: **I am open to receiving good advice.**

CHAPTER

28

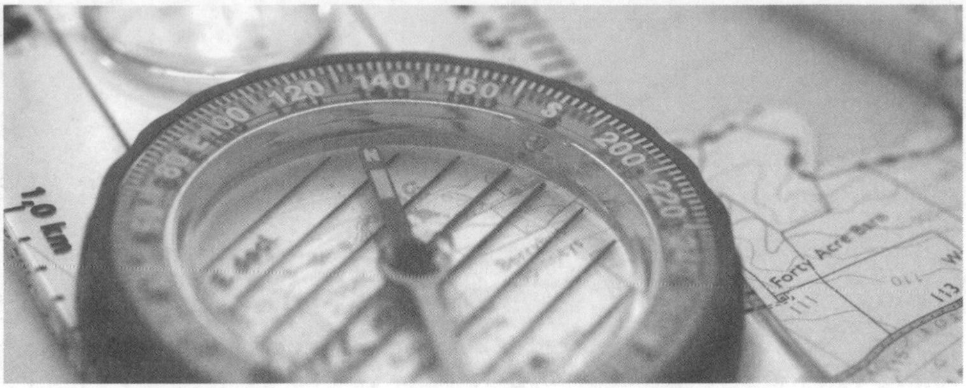

Your Automobile

The successful man is the one who finds out what is wrong with his business before his competitors do.

—Roy L. Smith

Are you using your car as an advertising tool, not to mention a tax deduction? You can get vanity plates with your business name on them, or just a plate holder, if you can't fit your name on the plate itself. It's relatively inexpensive to have professional lettering put on your car—or go the cheap route like I did and do it yourself! I purchased a set of vinyl letters for less than five dollars and just put the name of my business and the phone number on the back window. A well-known sports massage therapist, teacher, and author I know from our state has "Over 40,000 massages given" in big letters on his car. You can't help but notice it. If your car is leased, and you can't put permanent lettering on it, you could still put magnetic signs on at a reasonable cost, or a vanity tag. And remember, if you do outcalls, your car is more or less your office. Keep it clean!

My Story

Adrienne's Story

I purchased a set of magnetic signs to put on my mini-van doors for less than a hundred dollars, and sometimes when I'm sitting at a stoplight I can see the person next to me writing down my number. I also have the AMTA decal on my back window, and a plate holder that says "Hire a Professional Massage Therapist." I strictly do outcalls and use a cell phone as my business phone. Often, as I am at leaving someone's house after doing a massage, I'll have a message that says something like, "I saw your van at the Smith's on Pine Street. I'm at 424 Maple just around the corner and wondered if you had time to do another massage while you're in the neighborhood. My number is 555-9898." If I can't take care of them right then, I still have the chance to make a future appointment with them. That wouldn't happen if I wasn't using my car to advertise my services.

Beware the IRS

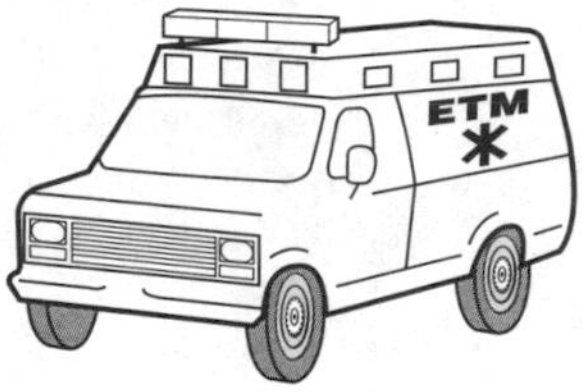

Remember, your car is not a tax deduction on the whole, unless it is utilized only for your business. Of course, there are allowable deductions for using your personal car for business purposes. The IRS website, www.irs.gov, can clarify what is deductible and what is not. For instance, therapists who make a living doing house calls have special circumstances. If you have no regular office, and you do not have an office in your home, the location of your first business contact is considered your office. Transportation expenses between your home and this first contact are nondeductible commuting expenses. Transportation expenses between your last business contact and your home are also nondeductible commuting expenses. Although you cannot deduct the costs of these trips, you can deduct the costs of going from one client or customer to another.

If your principal place of business is your home, but you make on-site calls, you can deduct the round-trip cost to the client's home or office. Travel to attend work-related conventions, seminars, board meetings, and Continuing Education classes is also tax deductible.

Expenses related to the business use of your automobile, whether it is used for advertising purposes or strictly for transportation, are best discussed with a tax professional. The wisdom of whether to take the standard mileage deduction or whether to keep track of actual expenditures may hinge on several things such as whether your car is leased or owned; that also has an effect on depreciation of the vehicle. It's safest to consult a tax professional before making any decisions. As a taxpayer and business person, you want to get the maximum tax benefits you are entitled to—while at the same time getting the maximum amount of exposure for your business at the lowest cost possible.

If your car is a new Corvette, you probably don't want to use it as an advertising tool—and you probably don't need to worry about cheap ways to advertise, either!

My Personal Journey

This Week's Activity: Utilizing my Automobile Date ____________

For this week's activity, you are going to make certain that you are using your automobile in the best possible way for the benefit of your business. If you are willing to use your car for advertising, look into having lettering or a magnetic sign put on your car. If you prefer not to use your car as an actual advertising tool, spend time on the IRS website or with a tax professional to find out exactly how you can benefit tax-wise through the business use of your automobile and start your record-keeping.

My Goals

___

___

___

What's in my way?

___

___

___

What action can I take to remedy the situation?

___

___

___

One-Year Progress Update Date ____________

___

___

___

POSITIVE AFFIRMATION: **My car will take me safely wherever I go.**

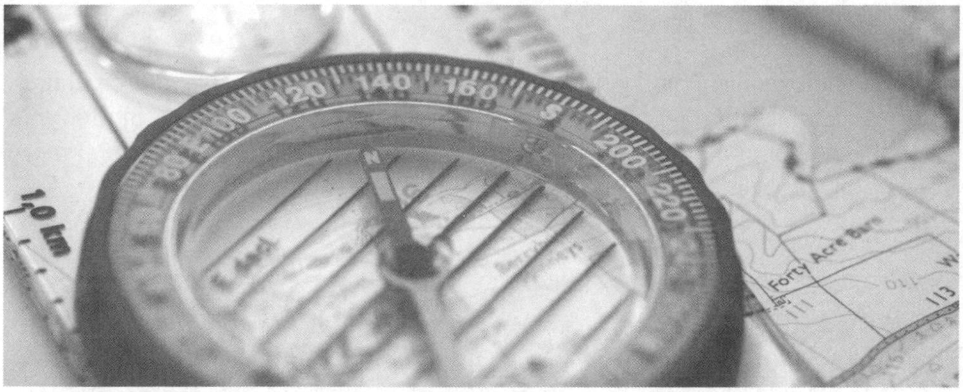

CHAPTER 29

Bartering for Advertising

Success is more a function of consistent common sense than it is of genius.
—AN WANG

Bartering is one of the oldest concepts in the world. You have something someone needs, they have something you need, and you agree to make a trade. One caveat—the Internal Revenue Service would like for you to pay taxes on bartered goods, just the same as if it had been a cash transaction. Remember you heard it here!

Where to Barter

A big-city, syndicated newspaper is probably not in a position to barter with you for advertising space. Small-town papers, regional magazines and papers, local cable channels, locally owned radio stations, and those type places are much more approachable. I've traded gift certificates with all the above for promotional give-aways in exchange for free ads. There are so many more marketing opportunities that you could barter for:

- A Web designer could upgrade your homemade website to something really snazzy.
- A graphic designer could get you beautiful and professional-looking business cards, brochures, and other business literature.
- A printer could get you custom invoices, flyers, and other items you might need reproduced.
- A marketing genius could get you more brilliant ideas, in addition to what we've covered in this book.
- Someone who sells promotional items could get you giveaways for your clients with your name printed on them.
- An interior designer could get your office spruced up. Make it someone who knows *feng shui*, and they'll look after the energy flow, too.
- A restaurant or caterer could get you nice food for your open house or grand opening.

- A photographer could get you nice pictures for your advertising or brochures.
- A sign maker could get you a nice sign for your office, or lettering for your front door or automobile.
- A press agent could get you media attention.

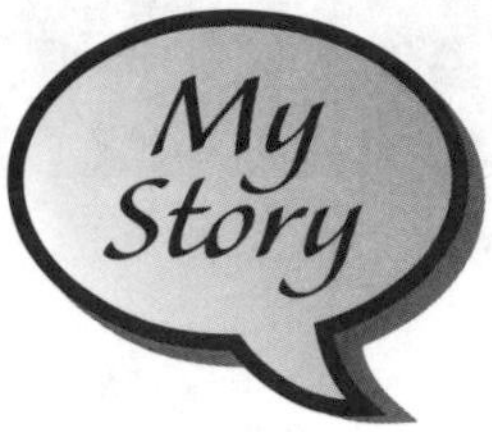

Kiki's Story

I was fortunate enough to obtain a nice office at a good price courtesy of a relative who owns the professional building it's located in. I felt it was important to have a nice sign, and the estimate was almost $1,000, more than I could afford. On an impulse, I asked the owner of the sign company to barter for massage, and he immediately took me up on it. I agreed to give him one massage per month for a year. I have a great sign: he's happy, and I'm happy. He's also sent me several other clients. It never hurts to ask for a barter—the answer might be yes!

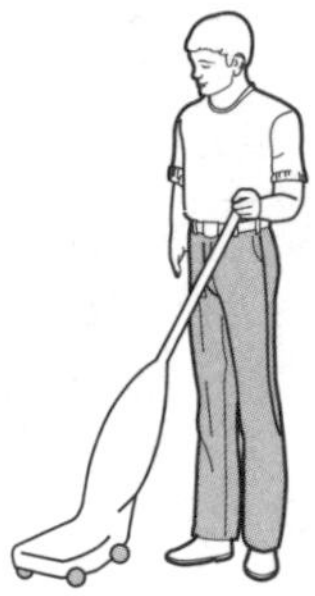

Of course, you can barter for other things you need besides marketing. I barter for having the carpets cleaned in my office every other month. You can barter for landscaping, having the lawn mowed, or the leaves raked, repairs to your office, laundry service, and virtually anything else you need. There are Internet bulletin boards, "swap-n-shop" papers devoted to bartering, or you could place a cheap classified ad stating you are willing to trade massage for so-and-so. Someone will take you up on it! I accidentally wound up on a website for a college bulletin board the other day, and at least half the kids on it were asking for massage—and offering everything in exchange from babysitting, running errands, typing services, altering clothes to guitar lessons. Ask and you shall receive!

I must include a few words to the wise about bartering. If you enter into a bartering relationship with someone, it is important to keep a check on the relationship to make sure both parties are happy with the arrangement. Things could go awry if one person doesn't uphold their end of the bargain, and you certainly don't want anger and resentment to enter into a relationship with either friend or business associate. Some therapists refuse to barter altogether because of past experiences that didn't turn out right. This is particularly true of relationships you may have with other therapists for trading massage. Do your part to keep the balance if you have such an arrangement with someone, and the minute you start to perceive that things are unbalanced, don't stew about it; talk about it without letting shame and blame enter into the conversation.

My Personal Journey

This Week's Activity: Bartering

Date ____________________

For this week's activity, you are going to learn to barter to get free advertising and other goods and services that you need. Start by making a list of media outlets that you could approach with a bartering proposal in exchange for advertising—and then approach them. Then make a list of other goods and services that you would be willing to barter for. Make flyers and hang them around town, advertise it on your website, or take out a cheap classified ad announcing your willingness to barter massage therapy in exchange for the advertising and other things you need. Chances are there are business people right in your neighborhood you could barter with; start there.

My Goals

___

___

___

What's in my way?

___

___

___

What action can I take to remedy the situation?

___

___

___

One-Year Progress Update

Date ____________________

___

___

___

POSITIVE AFFIRMATION: **My barters are always fair exchanges.**

CHAPTER

30

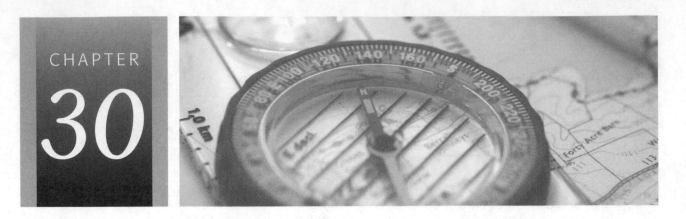

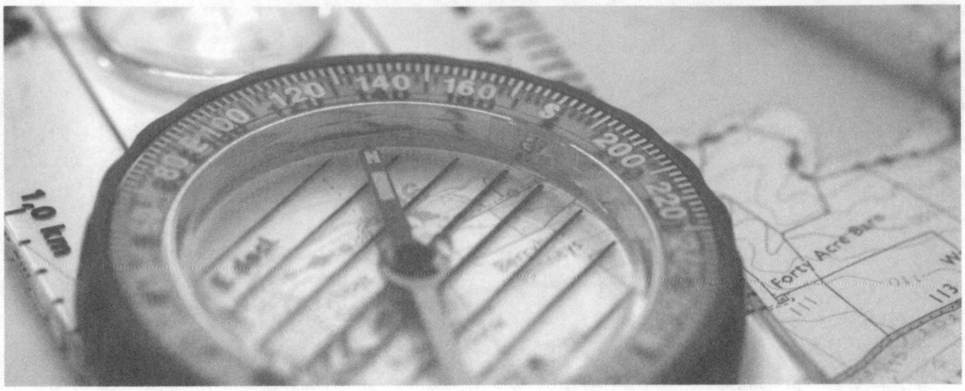

Retailing

Success in business requires training and discipline and hard work. But if you're not frightened by these things, the opportunities are just as great today as they ever were.

—David Rockefeller

Retailing items in your massage therapy office can be a double-edged sword, but it can also be a very lucrative source of income if you handle it correctly. When I say double-edged sword, I am referring to the fact that acting as a retailer, as well as a massage therapist, puts you in the position of assuming dual roles, a situation therapists usually try to avoid. If you will remember that you are first and foremost a massage therapist, not a salesman, and never tell a client that they "need" or "must have" something that you are retailing, you'll be fine.

Choosing the Right Items to Retail

The first items I purchased to retail in my office were hot/cold packs that could be put in the microwave or the freezer. That way, when I advise someone to use ice or heat—there they are, and they're cheap, too. Because I buy them in bulk, I get them for a little more than a dollar, and sell them for three—almost a 200% markup. You can even go all out and get some imprinted with your name or your business name and contact information on them.

I have been in the offices of other massage therapists who were selling jewelry, books and CDs, crystals, and any number of things. I am not criticizing them, and it may be bringing in a lot of money. I have personally chosen to sell only things that relate to massage and bodywork and the other services we offer here, and that seems to work well. My retail items include pillows, topical creams, lotions, essential oils, hot/cold packs, organic herbal salves, and ear coning supplies. The salt glow, mud, and lotions we use in our spa services can also be purchased for home use. I also have a line of organic botanical skincare products that our aesthetician uses for facials. I had not really considered selling those items, but when customers began to ask if they could buy the products we were using on them to take home, I accommodated them.

Boyd's Story

Since my business is outcalls, I really never intended to retail any products, but it seemed with every massage people were interested in the essential oils I used on them. I just started by carrying a few extra bottles with me and selling them (only when they asked, I never solicit anyone). It's a nice little supplement to my income.

At various times, I have tried retailing herbs and supplements, and a line of all-natural mineral makeup, which did not personally work for me, but I know others who have done quite well at it. You will have to find what works for you, basically through trial and error. Try to avoid dealing with any companies that require you to make a big minimum order. It's better to get stuck with $50 worth of product than it is to get stuck with $500 worth of product.

I had quite a few products from one particular company that were not moving, even after I put them on sale, so I made a very grand-looking gift basket for Valentine's Day and had a drawing for a free basket of natural beauty products. It was a tax write-off for me, I got rid of the stuff that was taking up space, and the winner was thrilled with the basket.

Many therapists just starting out are not in a cash flow position to lay out a lot of money for retail items. Don't go into debt to retail. Avoid the temptation to max out a credit card buying retail items. Start out slowly with just a few items. It's also nice to find dealers who will let you sell items on consignment. I sell a line of organic herbal salves that are handled in just that manner. The dealer comes in once a month, I pay him for what's been sold, and he restocks the shelves.

Another thing to consider with retailing is giving out samples of the items you retail. For instance, one of the topical creams that we use can be purchased in a box of 100 sample packs at a cost of about 25 cents per pack. The retail size of the product sells for about $10. By giving away the sample packs so people can try it, I sell a lot of the full size product. I also sell a lot of essential oils by giving samples. I purchase the tiny vials that perfume samples come in and just give people a few drops of the oil. Many times, they come back to buy the bottle.

Before jumping into retailing, remember that most states require you to have a resale license and a tax identification number, and that you will have to pay retail sales tax on the items you sell. It's also wise to let your stock run down as far as possible near the end of the year, as you will have to pay tax on any inventory you have on hand. If you have any doubts about the situation in your particular state, give a call to your state department of revenue or local small business office and they'll be able to tell you what's expected of you.

Retailer for a Day

One strategy that I recently started taking advantage of is akin to that old time-tested concept, the Tupperware party. This came about when a friend of mine stopped in all excited to show me her new bra. Yes—she was very excited about a bra. It seems that Oprah Winfrey had recently done a show about this particular brand of bra, which is sold only through home parties. We all know that Oprah can say the word and whatever she's talking about will instantly become the next big thing or best seller, right? This bra was no exception.

I called the distributor who made the offer to give me free products in exchange for holding one of her bra parties here. Then I sent an email blast to our female clients saying we were having a personal bra fitter at the office for the day. I am still reeling from the shock when I say that 39 women paraded through here in one long day to get fitted for a bra. I never imagined the response we would get. In addition to a very grand amount of free stuff, I also had the benefit of several of our women clients bringing in friends who had never been here before, who ended up booking massage and aesthetic services while they were here.

The next thing I held was a skin care party. Only six women attended—and those six women spent over $2,000—more nice products for me to use (or sell, if I don't care for them personally). It went so well I decided to become a distributor and retail the line in my office, as well as having our aesthetician use it for facials, and it's still selling well more than a year later. Having different distributors come in with their goods can be a way to stick your toe in the water for selling things at your office. The jewelry, the make-up, the crystals, and other things I don't want to invest in might be a great draw for a one-day show. An art show could be a good sales promotion, especially if you could have the artist present. They could show their work, meet your customers, and give you 30% commission on what they sell. If you announce your retail promotions ahead of time, the people who do have an interest will show up, and there's no pressure on anyone to buy; tell them they're of course welcome to just look.

My Personal Journey

This Week's Activity: Retailing Date ____________________

For this week's activity, you are going to research retailing products to complement your business. Even if you do not intend to retail at this time, do the research so you'll have an idea of what's out there that might appeal to your clients. Keep in mind that they may especially want to purchase the products that you use with them during massage. If you know you want to retail, go ahead and get the necessary licenses or permits you need. And if you are already retailing, take a look at what you could do to increase your sales—even something as simple as rearranging your shelves so that things look more attractive or advertising products on your website.

My Goals

____

____

____

What's in my way?

____

____

____

What action can I take to remedy the situation?

____

____

____

One-Year Progress Update Date ____________________

____

____

____

POSITIVE AFFIRMATION: **I am grateful for the extra income I receive from retailing.**

CHAPTER

31

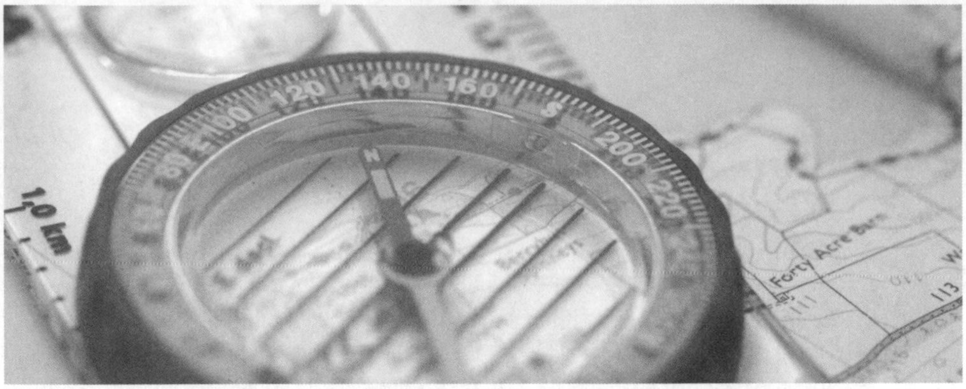

Everybody Loves a Parade

Eighty percent of success is showing up.

—Woody Allen

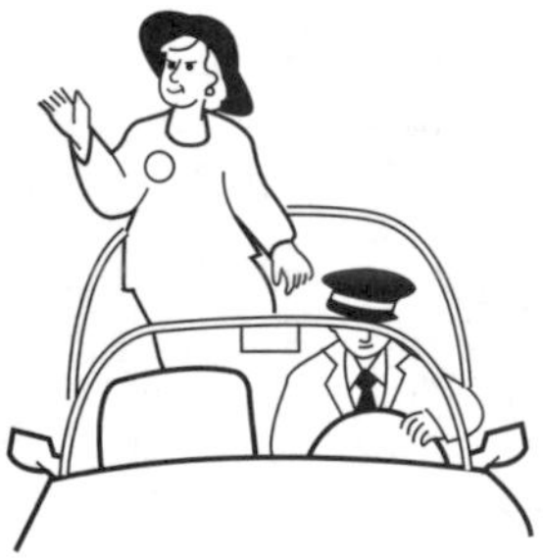

People love parades. Almost every town has a parade at one time or another throughout the year, a Christmas parade, Veteran's Day, Founder's Day, or some other occasion. Participating in a parade can expose your business to hundreds of people at once.

Parade Possibilities

Most high schools have a Homecoming parade and a Health Occupations class. Offer to sponsor a float for the class in the homecoming parade in exchange for having your business name on the float. The cost of the sponsorship will be decorating the float and a couple of printed signs or posters with your business name on it—not a lot. Of course, you can get as fancy as you can afford. If you're not the creative type, enlist someone who is to help you.

If your town holds a parade, they probably actively search for businesses willing to sponsor floats. Call your Chamber of Commerce or merchant's association for details. You don't even have to have a float. Recruit a friend with a classic car or hot rod, to drive you in the parade, or just walk. As you walk or ride through the parade, pass discount coupons out to the crowd.

Street festivals are also popular in towns and cities of every size. Within a 20-mile radius of my business is the annual Mayfest (right up the street), several Octoberfests, an Apple Festival, a Peach Festival, Coon Dog Days, a Cool Rides festival showcasing antique and classic cars, and several more. Set up a massage chair and be prepared to be busy all day, if you participate in something like this. You can do this for community service, or charge a dollar a minute for your own coffers or for charity, if you're led to do that. Take plenty of business cards and brochures along with you. In the two festivals in my town that I annually participate in, on the average myself and a couple of other therapists from my office will do a chair massage on close to two hundred people in a day. Many more stop by the booth just to watch and to enter the drawing for the free hour of massage we give away.

Juanita's Story

My dad has a vintage Corvette and belongs to a classic car club. They're always participating in parades, festivals, and car shows. I always rent a booth and offer chair massage during these events. They're usually on a weekend, when my office is closed anyway, and at a dollar a minute, plus tips, I can easily make five hundred dollars in a day and have fun while I'm doing it. I always have cards and brochures with me. If it's a local event, I'm bound to get new customers out of it, and even when the event is somewhere out of town, the potential is still there to meet people who visit your town or have friends or relatives there for whom they might buy gift certificates.

In the same spirit is the annual fireworks display on the fourth of July. Our town asks for sponsors, and if you are a sponsor, you are heavily advertised (at the Chamber's expense) in every ad that mentions the fireworks. It's a good value for the money because of the repetitive ads, and you don't have to spend a fortune to participate. It's also a good way to give the perception that *you* are a civic-minded individual who supports your community, always a good thing when it comes to business. They're also photo opportunities.

The local newspapers always cover parades and street festivals—and they might photograph *you.* At a minimum, the participating sponsors usually get a free mention or two in the paper. Even if they don't, it's a great way to get a massive amount of exposure. A parade is a great excuse to get out of the office, have a little fun, and publicize your business all in one fell swoop.

My Personal Journey

This Week's Activity: Participating in a Parade Date ____________________

Chances are there may not be a parade this particular week—and if not, that's okay—you can use the time to contact your local high schools, Chamber of Commerce, Merchant's Association, or Town Council to find out when the next one is going to take place. Securing a spot in a parade only takes a minute. Planning your participation will take substantially longer. Write up a plan. Are you going to have a float, walk among the crowd, or ride in a classic car? Decorating a float can take minutes or weeks, depending on how fancy you get. Are you going to pass out literature? Will you have a particular theme, such as "Massage Reduces Stress"? After you sign up to participate, formulate your plan and get ready to showcase your business in front of hundreds or thousands of people lining Main Street.

My Goals

___

___

___

What's in my way?

___

___

___

What action can I take to remedy the situation?

___

___

___

One-Year Progress Update Date ____________________

___

___

___

POSITIVE AFFIRMATION: **I am a welcome addition to any event I participate in.**

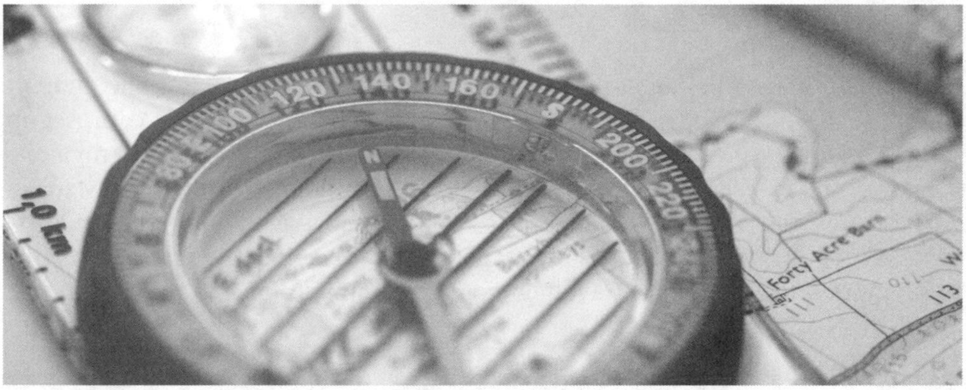

CHAPTER 32

Have Table, Will Travel

Much of the success of life depends upon keeping one's mind open to opportunity and seizing it when it comes.

—Alice Foote MacDougall

How about a business with hardly any overhead? If you decide to cultivate a business doing Outcalls, that's what you'll have. Even if you work from an office, you can cultivate Outcalls if you like, but that's part of the beauty of Outcalls—you don't need your own workspace. A cell phone, a massage table, oils and linens, and transportation are the only things you really need.

Set Your Parameters

Marketing Outcalls is a simple thing, but you will want to set some ground rules first. You're going to have to decide what you are comfortable with. For example, you may want to cultivate Outcalls at the Ritz, or the Hilton on the Harbor, but not at the Trucker's Paradise on the bypass. You may choose not to go to the homes (or guest accommodations) of people of the opposite sex unless they have been personally recommended to you by an existing client you know and trust. You may only want to go in the daytime, not at night; you may choose to go to bed and breakfasts, but no hotels at all. If you specialize in geriatric massage, you may do a lot of calls at rest homes or assisted living facilities. There are so many opportunities. You may only want to go a certain radius away from your home, mileage-wise.

The Price Is Nice

Once you have decided what you are willing to do, you'll need to decide how to price your services. You may want to charge extra for going a certain distance. Going across town takes more of your time than going a mile away, and in addition to your skill, that's what you're charging for—your time. Alternatively, you can charge mileage instead of a flat rate, and inform the client beforehand that it will be added to the price of the massage.

Outcalls are worth more money than in-house appointments. For one thing, it doesn't matter if it's across the street, by the time you lug everything over, set up and break down, you could have done two appointments in the office. In my area, the going rate for massage in-house is $50 to $60 per hour (barring a fancy spa at a nearby resort that charges $250 for a 50-minute massage, and you would be appalled at how little of that goes to the therapist). The going rate for an Outcall is $100; more if the therapist is traveling more than ten miles or so.

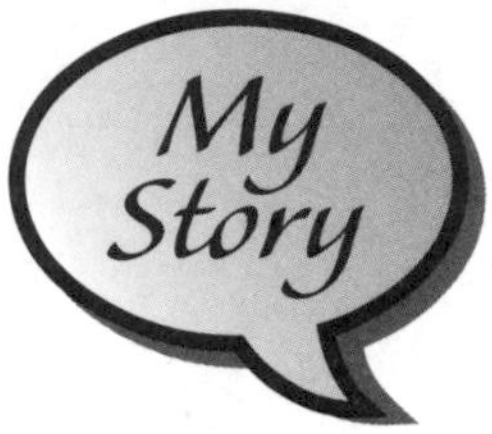

Pamela's Story

I strictly do house calls, and I wouldn't have it any other way. I live near a lakeside resort community with a lot of rental properties, Bed-and-Breakfasts, and hotels, and my cards and brochures are in as many of them as I can get them in. I earn enough money from spring to fall to take the winter months off.

Once you have decided on all the particulars, you'll need business cards and brochures advertising your services—and then take the time to place them where they'll do the most good. For example, if you are willing to go to hotels (and I advise that you stick to the high-end ones), approach the manager and ask if you may leave brochures in the lobby, at the desk, or in the rooms. Make it plain to them that you strictly practice therapeutic massage; go armed with your license in hand, and your professional-looking business literature, dressed like the professional you are. A nice hotel is not going to display tacky-looking printed materials; this is one time not to skimp on costs. The hotel could also reasonably ask you for a percentage of what you make, but that is between you and them, and should be discussed at the initial meeting.

Other places to leave your brochures are at Bed-and-Breakfasts. Couples' massage is very popular at B & B's in our area. If you have a fellow therapist who's willing to accompany you, it's a great service to offer, especially at the romantic-type places that cater to honeymooners, if you're near a resort or tourist area.

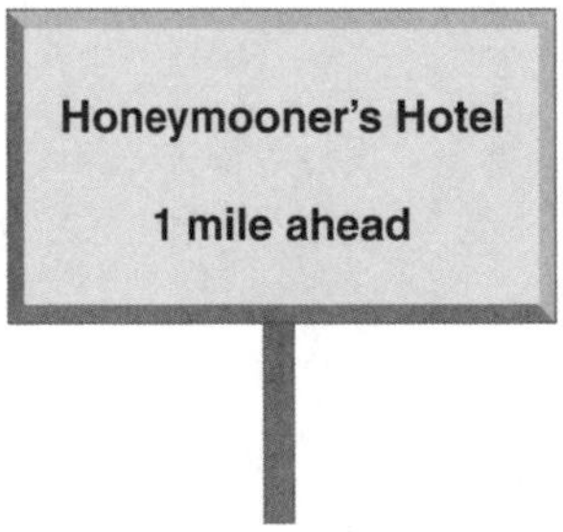

If you have developed referral relationships with physicians, be sure to let them know that you are willing to do Outcalls. They may have patients who are bedridden or temporarily unable to come out due to an injury, who would welcome an Outcall. If you have a good relationship with other therapists in your area who refuse to do Outcalls, let them know that you are willing to do them and provide them with some of your business cards and brochures.

Safety First

Your primary concern with Outcalls is always your personal safety. Keep your cell phone and keys on your body, not in your purse, at all times. When you arrive at the appointment, call someone and let them know where you are, and what time you will be calling them back to check in. At a hotel, tell the manager that when you receive a call to come to their establishment, that you will be stopping at the front desk and checking in, telling the person on duty what room you are going to, and asking that if you are not down by a specified time, that they send security to check on you. That is the professional way to handle it. Collect the money at the beginning of the session. Always follow proper draping procedures. If any suggestion of impropriety makes you uncomfortable, or if you feel threatened or uneasy in any way, just leave. Leave your table if you have to, and return with a friend or the police if necessary to retrieve it.

Outcalls are not for everybody, but if you decide to cultivate them, it can be very lucrative. At $100 per Outcall, you could do three appointments a day and call it a day. That's not bad money, and most people tip well for Outcalls, too. Another point to consider is that while you may not intend for your career in massage to be Outcalls forever, it is a good way to make money on a temporary basis without much overhead while you save up for that nice office you'd like to have.

My Personal Journey

This Week's Activity: Cultivating Outcalls Date ____________________

If you're still a student, chances are you're already doing a few Outcalls in the interest of practicing the massage techniques you're learning and meeting your practicum obligation. If you're a new therapist, Outcalls can help you get established, and can help pay the rent on your office. If you're an established therapist who's looking to revitalize their practice, you might consider adding some Outcalls onto your menu of services. It's your choice, of course, but remember, Outcalls will get you out of the office and meeting some new people, if nothing else. You could even partner with another therapist and offer couple's massage on an Outcall basis.

My Goals

____

____

____

What's in my way?

____

____

____

What action can I take to remedy the situation?

____

____

____

One-Year Progress Update Date ____________________

____

____

____

POSITIVE AFFIRMATION: **I enjoy going to new places and meeting new people.**

CHAPTER

33

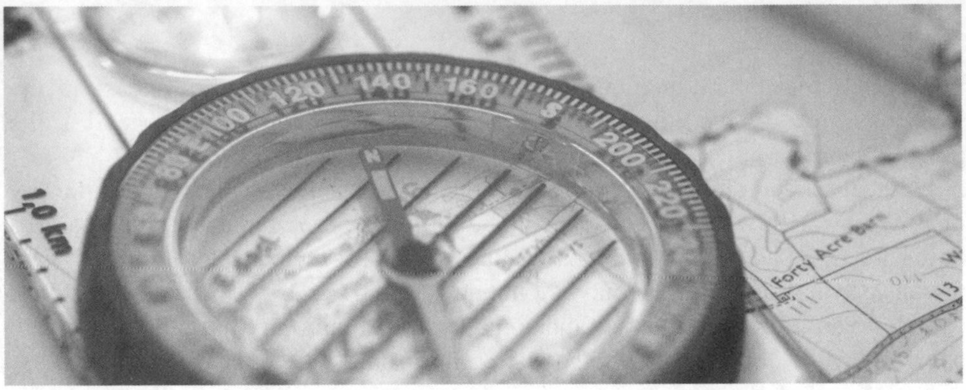

The Magnificent Massage Chair

The truth is that all of us attain the greatest success and happiness possible in life whenever we use our native capacities to their greatest extent.

—Dr. Smiley Blanton

A massage chair is one of the best investments you can make from a marketing standpoint. There is so much you can do with it, so many ways to get new customers and attention for your business. A chair is a lot less trouble to take out to community service events and festivals than a table. It's lightweight; you don't need linens. While you can spend close to $1,000 on a top-of-the-line chair, that's not necessary. I have purchased several from Internet auctions for around $130 each. It can pay for itself in no time. You can also purchase a breast pad/face cradle combination that sits on any table or desk. And when you need to, improvise. You can actually do a great chair massage with the person sitting in any kind of chair.

In the Office

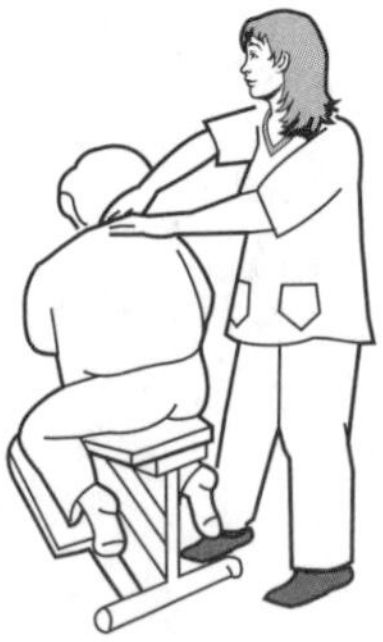

Has this ever happened to you—someone walks in the door and wants a massage right then; you can't accommodate them because you have someone else scheduled in half an hour? My massage chair sits in my lobby. Next to it is a sign advertising "The Stressbuster—15 minutes of seated massage for $15." It's a moneymaker! Sometimes, people come in to buy a gift certificate and decide to have one on the spot. And of course, if you can't do it right then, you can offer them another time. I also sell gift certificates for these, and they're very popular. People buy them for co-workers or someone they want to give a gift to but don't want to spend a lot. One chiropractor that I have a mutual referral relationship with purchases them for his clients—and of course, once they get the 15 minutes, they're ready to book a whole session. $15 doesn't seem like a lot of money, but over time it really adds up, and if you're just starting out and have a lot of downtime, it can make a big difference to your paycheck.

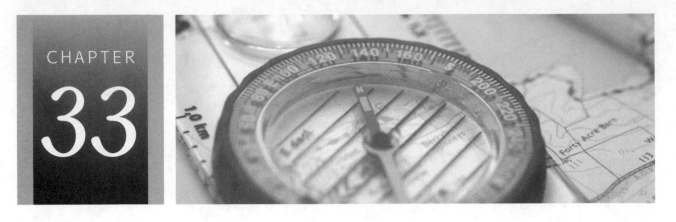

Corporate Chair Massage

Adding Corporate Chair Massage to your menu of offerings can be a very lucrative moneymaker for you—both in terms of what you'll get paid on the spot for doing it—and in terms of the people who will book an appointment after they've had a little taste of your chair massage.

Getting your foot in the door at a large factory is usually easiest if you approach the Human Resources Director first. Most factory general managers or owners are very busy people (just like you) who may not be inclined to take the time to listen to your sales pitch. Pitch it to the Human Resources person first—after all, she's already acquainted with the manager, so it won't be a cold call. She will probably have the inside track on persuading the company that they need your services.

There are actually two different ways to approach corporate chair massage days: (i) persuade the company to pay for it as an employee benefit (and don't fail to remind them that it's a tax write-off when you send your letter), or (ii) let the employees pay for their own.

A dollar a minute is the going rate for chair massage in my area. Let's say you do five people, ten minutes each, in an hour and have ten minutes for an hourly break. If you stay for an 8-hour workday, you've made $400, which may be less than you would have made in your office for a full day. However, you've met 40 potential new clients, something that would not have occurred at your office.

Below is a sample letter pitching corporate chair massage. Be sure to follow up with a phone call within a week or so.

Sample Letter for Corporate Chair Massage Proposal

Laura Allen, LMBT
THERA-SSAGE
431 S. Main St., Ste. 2
Rutherfordton, NC 28139

Ms. Betsy Mooney
The Pickle Factory
1000 Dill Dr.
Rutherfordton, NC 28139
01/17/2006

Dear Ms. Mooney,

My name is Laura Allen, and I am the owner of THERA-SSAGE Massage & Bodywork. As the Human Resources Director of a busy factory, I know that you are all too well familiar with the effects of stress in the workplace: on-the-job accidents, lost time, poor employee morale, and so forth, which leads to lowered productivity. One of the services that we offer is corporate chair massage, a great technique for relieving stress and improving the morale of your workers, which ultimately leads to better productivity in the workplace.

At the present time we are able to offer this service on your choice of Monday during any week of the month. We also have availability on the 3rd and 4th Fridays of the month.

This service may be provided by the company as an employee benefit, which of course is a tax deduction for the company, or you may have the employees who are interested pay for it themselves. The only thing we need is a space to work in, such as a break room or an unused meeting room.

I will be calling you within the next week to give you more details and to answer any questions you may have regarding this service. Thank you for your consideration, and I will look forward to speaking with you in person.

Sincerely,
Laura Allen

Be sure to make that follow-up phone call. Once you get your foot in the door in one place, it will be much easier to get the next one (you can always ask for client testimonials). It could also lead to bigger and better things. A former student of mine had only had his license for a couple of weeks, when he approached someone he was acquainted with who owns a manufacturing facility. He ended up getting put on a $1,500 per month retainer to be available eight hours a day, four days per month, not to mention getting a number of private clients out of the deal.

Cash Cow Lane

Doing corporate massage gives you a change of pace by getting you out of the office periodically and giving you the opportunity to meet lots of new people, as well.

Massage for Charity

A charity event is a great place to do chair massage, an opportunity for the public to get something in exchange for their donation, an opportunity for *you* to donate, and a marketing bonanza. While you're doing chair massage for a dollar a minute, and giving the proceeds (or even half) to the charity, you are making a good impression as a benevolent business person who gives back to the community and meeting new people—all potential customers. Have plenty of your business cards and brochures on hand to give out.

Make it something fun, if you care to. A therapist I know did 24 hours straight of chair massage at a local radio station to raise money for hurricane victims. He took a ten minute break every four hours, but other than that, he kept it up for the whole 24 hours and raised several thousand dollars. People were caught up in the giving spirit and impressed with what he was doing, and some paid $5 or $10 a minute instead of the $1 a minute he was actually charging. The radio station made a festive occasion out of it, inviting people to come out and get the massage, regular updates about how long he had been at it, and so forth, and over the 24 hour period that he was there, his name and business were probably mentioned on the air at least 50 times. He got a massive amount of publicity and goodwill, and quite a few new clients in addition to his grand donation.

My Story

Chanel's Story

I've been making my living doing chair massage in a coffee house for the past five years. It's located on Main Street in a tourist town that's popular year-round. I give the owner 20% of what I make for letting me work there, and he doesn't even want to take that because I'm good for business. I set my own hours and make more money in two days than I used to make in a week in an office, and am constantly meeting new and interesting people from all over.

My Personal Journey

This Week's Activity: Marketing Chair Massage Date ____________

For this week's activity, make it a priority to get a massage chair if you don't have one. If you're still a student, you can use it at Community Service Events, and Practicum. If you're cultivating a business, compose a letter like the previously mentioned sample and send it to ten possible venues for Corporate Chair Massage. Follow up in a couple of weeks with a phone call to the Human Resources Director. Keep repeating this exercise until you have at least one corporate chair massage account—or as many as you want.

My Goals

____

____

____

What's in my way?

____

____

____

What action can I take to remedy the situation?

____

____

____

One-Year Progress Update Date ____________

____

____

____

POSITIVE AFFIRMATION: **My massage chair is a magnet for money.**

CHAPTER 34

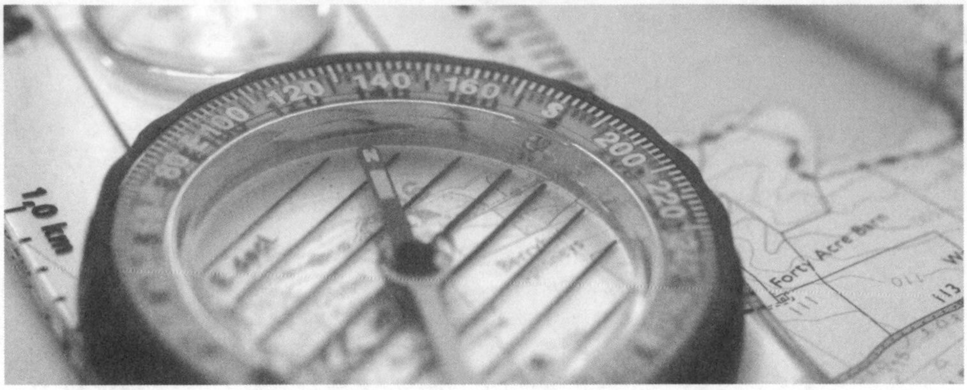

Adopt-a-Highway

There is only one success—to be able to spend your life in your own way.
—Christopher Morley

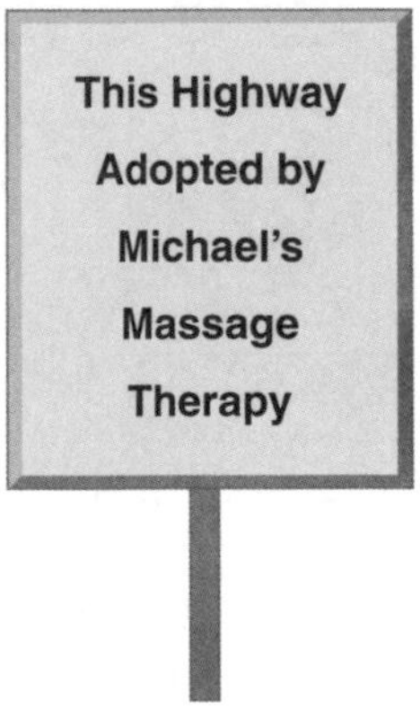

Nearly every state has an "Adopt-a Highway" or "Sponsor-a-Highway" program. Most require that you pick up litter along a two-mile stretch of the road between two and four times per year. In exchange for your efforts, you get a nice sign on the highway that says something like "The next two miles have been adopted by Michael's Massage Therapy." Just think about how many hundreds of people a day will drive past that sign, see the name of your business, and conclude that you are an environmentally conscious company.

In addition to the sign, you can also get inexpensive T-shirts with your company name and logo on them, and wear them while you are doing the trash pick-up. It's great if you can get the stretch of highway in front of your office, or as close to it as possible. If not, try to get a stretch of any nearby busy road or highway. Alternatively, you can sponsor a clean-up day for your street or your neighborhood, and offer discount coupons or give a chair massage to anyone who participates.

My Story

Bethany's Story

My husband's a chiropractor and we have an office together. We adopted the highway in front of our office and we try to clean it once a month. We're out there with our reflective vests on that we had lettered with our business name. I think people really appreciate our efforts because customers comment on seeing us out picking up trash, and several have even told me they made an appointment here because they saw us cleaning up the roadside.

You're making a contribution to a cleaner environment, getting a nice sign with your name on it out on the highway, and giving people the impression of a business that gives something back.

My Personal Journey

This Week's Activity: Adopt-a-Highway

Date ____________________

For this week's activity, contact the Highway Department to see about adopting a stretch of highway near your business. If you're not yet in business, you'll have that information for the future. If you work for someone else, do the legwork and then ask them to be the sponsor.

My Goals

____

____

____

What's in my way?

____

____

____

What action can I take to remedy the situation?

____

____

____

One-Year Progress Update

Date ____________________

____

____

____

POSITIVE AFFIRMATION: **Contributing to a clean environment is an enhancement to my business.**

CHAPTER

35

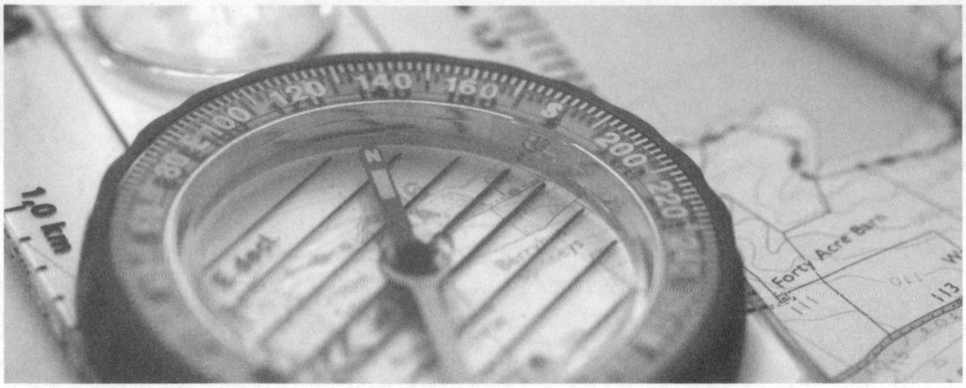

Host a Free Seminar

Aim for success, not for perfection. Never give up your right to be wrong, because then you will lose the ability to learn new things and to move forward with your life.

—Dr. David M. Burns

Hosting a free seminar is a great way to get people to come in and check out your business. You may not think of yourself as a public speaker, but if you stop and think about the things you deal with every day in your practice, you're probably somewhat of an authority on several things—not the least of which are the benefits of massage. Then there's fibromyalgia, carpal tunnel syndrome, stress, repetitive motion injuries in general, and any number of things that you can probably speak intelligently about. And you can always get a guest speaker.

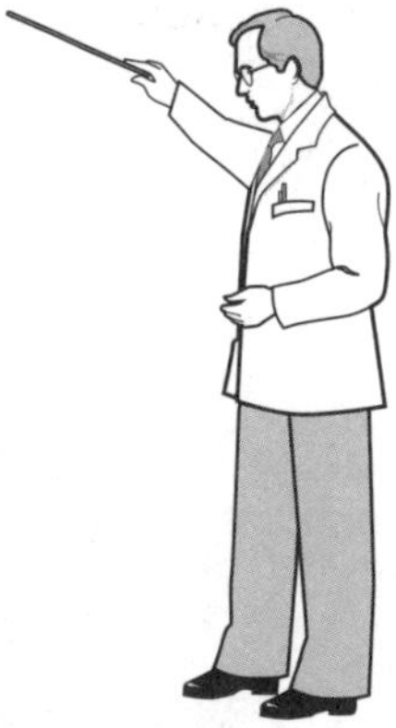

Get a Speaker

If you truly think you personally can't teach a seminar, ask a chiropractor or other health care professional you refer to if they would collaborate with you on a class. It doesn't have to be a seminar—you could host a support group for people who suffer from fibro, chronic fatigue syndrome, migraines, or any other condition you can think of. The first time I offered a seminar on "Living Well with Fibromyalgia," nine people came. That doesn't sound so great, but when you consider that only one of them had ever been here before, that means eight new people were exposed to my business. In addition to seminars on the benefits of massage for different conditions, you could also host a seminar on nutrition, stretching, exercise, or any other timely subject.

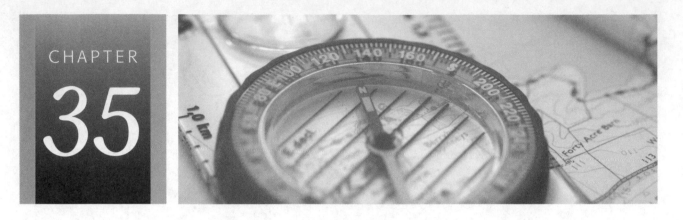

Martina's Story

My chiropractor agreed to come to my office and lead a presentation about osteoporosis. He offered free x-rays to every attendee who made a first-time visit to his office, and even gave me a free adjustment for having him there. Out of a dozen people who attended, four of them were people who hadn't been to my office before, and two made appointments with me in addition to almost everyone there taking him up on his offer. It turned out well for both of us and we plan to do it again.

If you are retailing any products, the company might send a representative to speak to your clients. A therapist I know sells flower remedies, and I attended a great seminar at her office a couple of years ago. Her office was packed full of interested people. The presenter gave everyone product samples on top of a lot of information about the remedies. People enjoyed it and many bought the products.

You might consider offering an incentive to your existing clients if they bring a guest who has never been to your office to the seminar.

If you don't have the space in your office to accommodate many people, you could use a church social hall, a community center, or some other cheap or free venue to hold it in. Be sure to take plenty of your business literature along to hand out. And, in addition to exposing new people to your business, you can usually get free advertising out of events like this. When you hold an event that's free and open to the public, send announcements to your local newspapers, radio stations, cable stations, and normally you will get put on the free public service announcements. I just type up something like the sample below and fax it to all the media outlets in my area. On the fax cover sheet, just write, "Please add this to your public service announcements." I haven't been turned down yet. The more venues you send it to, the more free publicity you are getting.

Public Service Announcement

Pinnacle Massage Therapy will be hosting a free seminar on Chronic Inflammatory Diseases on Monday, June 24 from 7 to 9 pm. The speaker will be Dr. Benjamin Deck, rheumatologist. Seating is limited. Call 288-3828 to reserve your free seat for the workshop.

My Personal Journey

This Week's Activity: Offer a Free Seminar

Date ____________________

For this week's activity, plan a free seminar. If you're still a student, you can start by gathering friends and family, and have them be your audience while you talk for at least thirty minutes on a subject related to massage. If you work in a chiropractor's office, you could collaborate on a seminar about massage and chiropractic working in harmony. If you're self-employed, lay your plans and then advertise the event with a two-week lead time. Hang a notice in your office, e-mail your clients. Keep it short, no longer than an hour. After all, it's free, and you don't want them to get *all* the information in one visit.

My Goals

____

____

____

What's in my way?

____

____

____

What action can I take to remedy the situation?

____

____

____

One-Year Progress Update

Date ____________________

____

____

____

POSITIVE AFFIRMATION: **My seminars serve the public and enhance my business.**

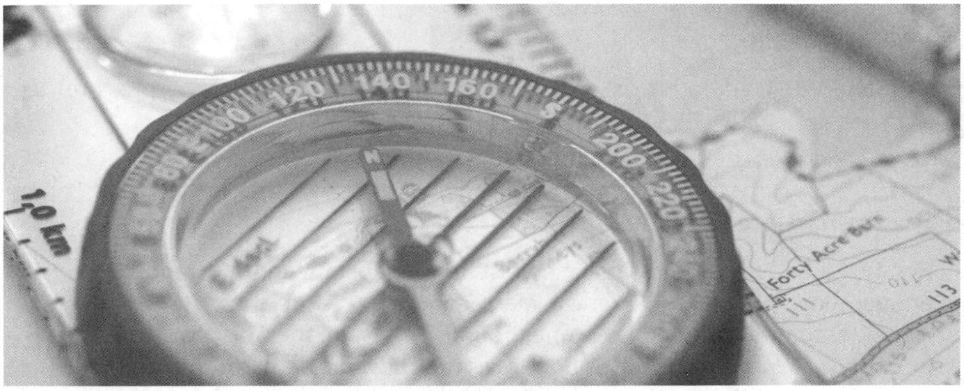

CHAPTER 36

Newsworthy Events and Press Releases

As a general rule the most successful man in life is the one who has the best information.

—Benjamin Disraeli

Opening a new business is of course a newsworthy event, one that most newspapers will cover at no cost. As mentioned in Chapter 35, hosting a free seminar can usually generate free advertising. Your objective is to get your name/business name in the news as many times as possible, at no cost to you. Press releases are the way to accomplish this. You may generate more newsworthy events than you realize. Don't overlook your graduation from massage school as being worth a press release—it certainly is! Most newspapers periodically run news about education—who's graduated from college or military boot camp. You're just as important. Here's a sample:

For Immediate Release

Richard Cavanaugh of Singleton has recently graduated from the 750-hour massage and bodywork program at the Southern School of Massage in Marlborough, and has been licensed by the North Carolina Board of Massage and Bodywork Therapy. Richard is working in the chiropractic offices of Dr. Leo Bushmill on Trade Street in Singleton. A native of Singleton, Richard graduated from Singleton Community College with a degree as a physical therapy assistant before pursuing the massage diploma. He is the son of Rev. and Mrs. John Cavanaugh of Singleton. He resides in the Woodbury community with his wife Cary and their son, Cody.

Stop the Press!

Have you attended any Continuing Education lately? Been to a state or national convention? Won an award? Had something published? That's newsworthy. Don't be shy about tooting your own horn. When you are submitting to the newspaper in particular, you should address your release to the business editor. A press release might look something like this:

For Immediate Release

Bonita Davis, Licensed Massage Therapist from Augusta, recently attended the annual convention of the American Massage Therapy Association (AMTA) in Albuquerque, New Mexico. Over one thousand massage therapists were in attendance. While at the convention, Davis took advanced classes in Orthopedic Massage, a modality that is very helpful to anyone who is recovering from a traumatic bone or other injury. Davis is an active volunteer in the Georgia chapter of AMTA and serves as the director of school relations on their behalf. She is the owner of The Body Temple on 2nd Street in Augusta.

There are other opportunities. If another therapist joins your practice, if you move to a new location, if you suddenly start offering a service that hasn't previously been available, or get a media appearance, let the public know. Here's another example:

For Immediate Release

Heather Nelon of Forest City, a Licensed Massage Therapist, will be featured tonight at 7 pm on the "Carolina Country" television show on Channel 47. Nelon has been a massage therapist since 1985, and is appearing as a part of WNBW's series of reports on complementary and alternative medicine. Nelon is a graduate of The Massage Institute, and also has a BFA from Warren Wilson College. She and her husband, Joe, a physical therapist, own Bodyworks in Forest City.

Collaborate

Any time you can get other practitioners to collaborate with you in offering a public service to the community, that's worthy of a public service announcement. In the small town that I live in, those are always listed on the front page of the newspaper—a prime spot! Right after I opened my practice, our local hospital announced in the newspaper that they had received a grant to conduct a research project on high blood pressure, and how lifestyle changes could have positive effects. The article stated that the hospital was looking for different venues around the county where they could hold free blood pressure checks. Guess who was the first one to call them? Right! The result of that has been that every six months, the hospital personnel come to my office for the free checkups—and *they* pay to advertise it. It appears in the newspaper, on the radio, and on the local cable channel, all at no cost to me. People file in and out of the office all day to get their free health checks. I don't have to do anything other than provide the hospital a corner of the office to set up their table and chair. They even put up a big sign right outside the office to attract walk-in clients. Since it's free and the hospital is co-sponsor, the media is glad to cover it in their public service announcements; the same applies to the free seminars mentioned in Chapter 35. Take advantage of any opportunities for free publicity that come your way—or that *you* create.

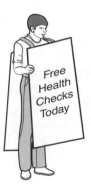

Get the Word Out

Writing the press release is only the first step. You have to get the word out. You should create a file for yourself with the names, addresses, phone and fax numbers, and contact information of all media outlets in your area—radio stations, newspapers, regional publications, television stations. Since these are public arenas, they'll be glad to give you their fax numbers and e-mail addresses to which you should send your announcements. Don't overlook any publication, no matter how small. In our area, there's a hokey little free paper that's distributed all over the county; it's full of satire about the local politicians and newsworthy events like who grew the biggest squash this year—and it's distributed free to 20,000–30,000 people a week. A town next to ours has the novel claim to fame that theirs is the smallest daily newspaper in America—it's $8\frac{1}{2}$ by 11—more than one page of course, and their advertising rates are very reasonable—but remember, you're going for free press. When you're planning events that you want announced ahead of time, be sure to give plenty of lead time for them to announce it—at least a few weeks. If you're sending out an announcement about something that's already happened, such as your attendance at a convention and so forth, be prepared for it to take a few weeks to make it into print, as those types of items are usually run on a first-come, first-served basis.

Visiting Media Outlets

It's happened often that someone interrupted my work day to try to sell me advertising. I have found a great way to nip that in the bud—and to increase my chances of getting free press—by going around and introducing myself. Particularly if you are new in business, this is a great strategy. Take your list of media outlets, and make time to visit each one in person. Armed with cards and brochures, go into the newspaper office and say you'd like to see someone about advertising. You don't have to be there to place an ad (and you don't have to make an appointment; after all, they don't make one when coming to you). Tell them you're gathering information for your future advertising campaigns. Introduce yourself, tell them the highlights of your business, and ask for an advertising rate sheet—which is, after all, information that you'll want to have. You are going to do *some* advertising, and you're covering your bases. Tell them that since you work on an appointment basis, you may not have time to see a sales rep who just pops into your business, but you are interested in what rates and package deals they have to offer. Give them a business card, and ask that the rep call you before coming by. Now you're not just a name to this person; you're a face, too. They'll be more apt to help you with free press when you send something in.

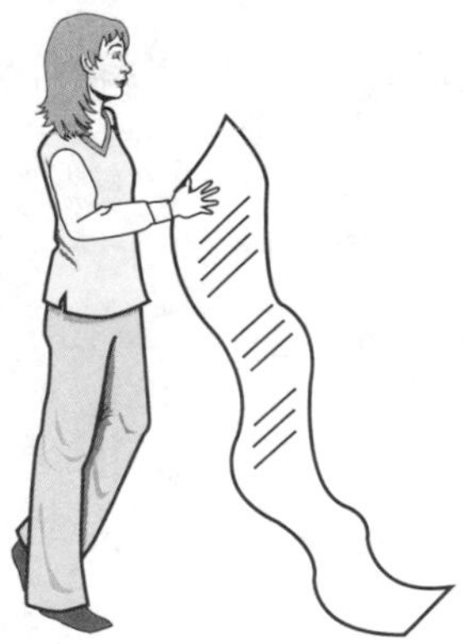

Zeke's Story

I try to get free publicity by way of a public service announcement or a press release every single month—that's my goal, and I usually meet it. I really enjoy going to the conventions, take a lot of Continuing Ed, doing things like holding free health checks at the office. Those things are all news in my local paper—as long as I send them in, and I do it religiously. Another therapist even commented to me that she sure did see my name in the paper a lot, and it sounded like she was slightly jealous. But if I don't blow my own horn, who will? I intend to get all the advertising I can without paying a penny for it.

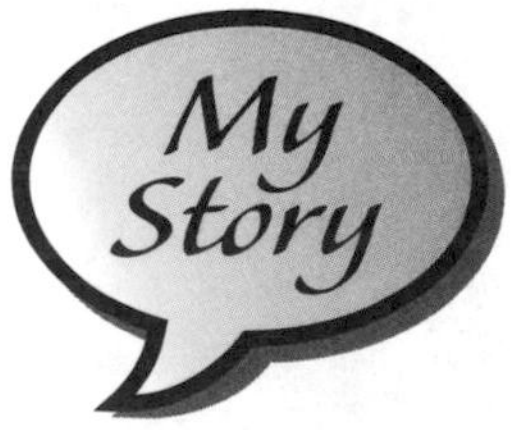

My Personal Journey

This Week's Activity: Getting Free Press Date ____________________

For this week's activity, you are going to write a press release. If you're still a student, prepare the release announcing your graduation. If you're established, make a list of the newsworthy things that have happened or are about to happen—new skills, a new therapist joining you, new services, convention attendance, and so forth. Create your media outlet file by obtaining the contact information for all the media outlets in your area and send something out. Keep a section of the file for your releases, and always keep copies of the media appearances you get.

My Goals

___

___

___

What's in my way?

___

___

___

What action can I take to remedy the situation?

___

___

___

One-Year Progress Update Date ____________________

___

___

___

POSITIVE AFFIRMATION: **I am worthy of all the positive publicity I can get.**

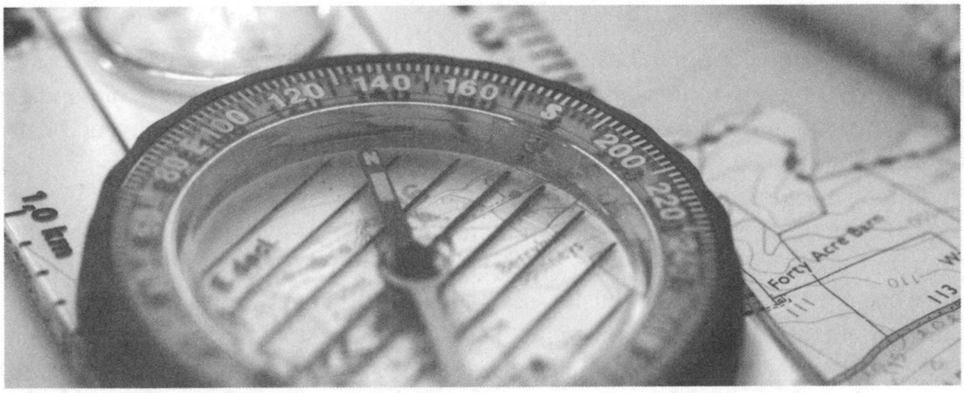

CHAPTER 37

Promotional Giveaways

We all have a few failures under our belt. It's what makes us ready for our successes.

—Randy K. Milholland

Everyone has a junk drawer in their house. Take a good look in yours. Among the pictures you've never put in the album, paper clips, pens that don't work, keys you no longer have any idea what they go to, and the other stuff you just can't seem to get around to throwing away, are probably lurking some promo items. You know what I mean: letter openers, key rings, tape measures, pill boxes, and so forth, with some company's name printed on them. Have any of them been useful to you? Probably not, or they wouldn't be residing in the junk drawer.

Giving Away the "Good" Goods

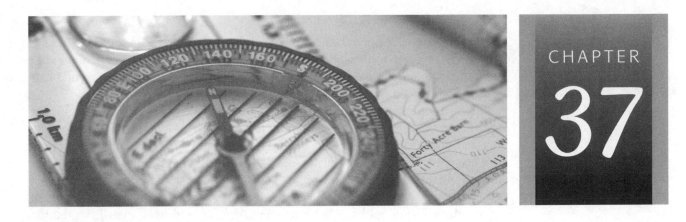

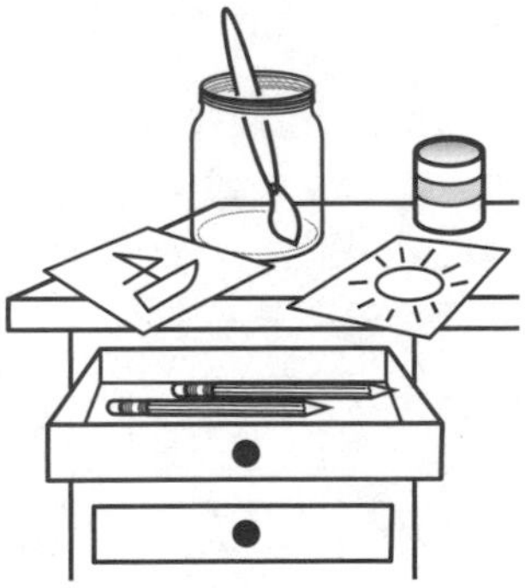

Putting your name on merchandise to give or sell to your clients can be a good marketing tool—or a total (and expensive) waste of money. If it's something you've thrown in your junk drawer instead of using it, don't buy it.

Consider the items I mentioned above. The tape measure, for instance. Now, that's a handy thing to have—once in a blue moon, unless you're a builder or a tailor. If you strictly cater to geriatric clients who tend to take a lot of prescription drugs, the pill box might be a great item for you. Letter openers are handy items, but how many do you need? Most people who want to use one already have one. They'll go in the junk drawer.

Clothing items such as t-shirts and caps usually won't be thrown away, but in reality, only select members of your clientele will wear them. Chances are they'll wind up at the goodwill store. A lot of men wear ball caps; most women won't. A lot won't wear t-shirts either; younger people seem to favor them, but middle-aged and up will not be out at the grocery store wearing your t-shirt. As the business owner, shirts or jackets with your name and logo on them for you and your staff members to wear may be a timely investment, but it's probably not wise to spend a lot of money on clothing items for clients who would only wear them once in a while, if at all. However, according to consumer research by www.promopeddler.com, a popular Internet company selling promotional items, wearable items such as shirts and hats are the most popular giveaways.

I recently turned down the opportunity to be advertised on a t-shirt with other local businesses. It was going to cost $500 for my business-card-size ad to be on one thousand shirts—and I would have been given 40 of the shirts. The remainder would have been distributed to other businesses. In reality, the shirts were something cheap that without the advertising, you could buy in any dollar store for a couple of bucks. Out of a thousand shirts that would be distributed, the chances are that on any given day maybe a few people would be wearing them around town, and I figured the possibility that anyone would get close enough to see my business card ad among a couple of dozen others was pretty slim. It didn't seem like a good deal to me. If the shirt only advertised my business and no one else's, it would have been more financially feasible for me, but still, I think there are better ways of spending my advertising dollars.

Refrigerator magnets are relatively inexpensive. Most people will take them home and stick them on the refrigerator—but they're not very handy if they usually call you from their office or their cell phone—again, a possible waste of money. Calendars and date books are nice. I probably received around 20 or 30 this year from various companies that I do business with, so there's a catch-22: exactly how many calendars does a person need, and will they use the ones from their favorite business, or one from their favorite charity, or whichever one is the prettiest or has the bigger space to write appointments in? It's hard to say. There are literally a million things you can have your name printed on, but if it's sitting in a drawer and not being used, it isn't worth the money you've spent on it.

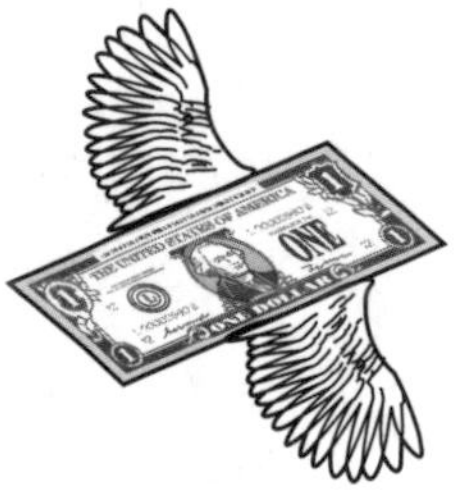

One thing that we all do as massage therapists is to encourage people to drink more water. Give them a water bottle on their way out. If it's a nice one, they'll keep it around. You can also get printed labels, or print your own, to stick on regular store-bought bottles of water if you give water to your clients. People won't throw away a nice coffee cup or travel cup, either.

We're in the business of getting people out of stress. Those little stress balls aren't very expensive, but I'm not sure they're not one of those items that winds up in the junk drawer; I've got several in mine. Pens are cheap, and the one item that most people use on a daily basis. You may want to use those as promo items, not only to give to clients, but as giveaways when you're working street festivals or community service events. Hot/cold packs can be cheaply imprinted with your name and make a nice giveaway to your clients at Christmas, for instance, but realistically the only people who will see them are your clients who are using them.

Tote bags make nice giveaways. They cost substantially more than a pen; but I have obtained nice ones for around $2 each when purchased in bulk. Environmentally conscious people use them all the time as shopping bags; others may use them as beach bags or book bags. If I am giving away a higher-end item like that, I will always ask the client if they could use one. Some folks turn me down, and say they have others at home they're not using, and that's fine. I want them to go to people who will get the most use out of them. After all, the point is for them to carry it around so others will see my business name on it.

Promotional items should serve two purposes: i) a gift to your clients and ii) a marketing tool to attract other clients. Be sure that any promo items you spend your advertising dollars on meet both those criteria.

Lester's Story

I have an office in a building with a lot of professionals and I have found that imprinted sticky notes are good promo items for me. Everybody in an office uses them, passes notes along to other people on them, and literally sticks them around!

My Story

My Personal Journey

This Week's Activity: Obtaining Promotional Items Date____________________

For this week's activity, you are going to research promotional items and fit them into your advertising budget. Check out some of the companies on the Internet that cater to our trade, or general promotional companies; there are literally thousands of them. Chances are there's a business in your town that sells promo items. Peruse the items for things that are useful and won't wind up in a drawer. Decide what you want and how many you can buy. If you're still a student or financially unable to purchase them right now, plan ahead for the day you'll be able to spend that money.

My Goals

____

____

____

What's in my way?

____

____

____

What action can I take to remedy the situation?

____

____

____

One-Year Progress Update Date____________________

____

____

____

POSITIVE AFFIRMATION: **My promotional items are a wise investment.**

CHAPTER

38

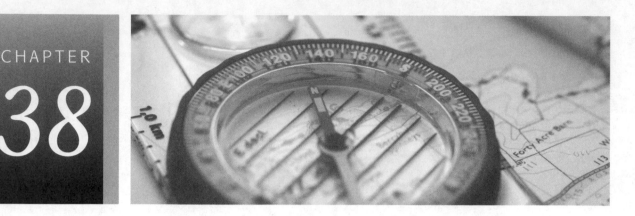

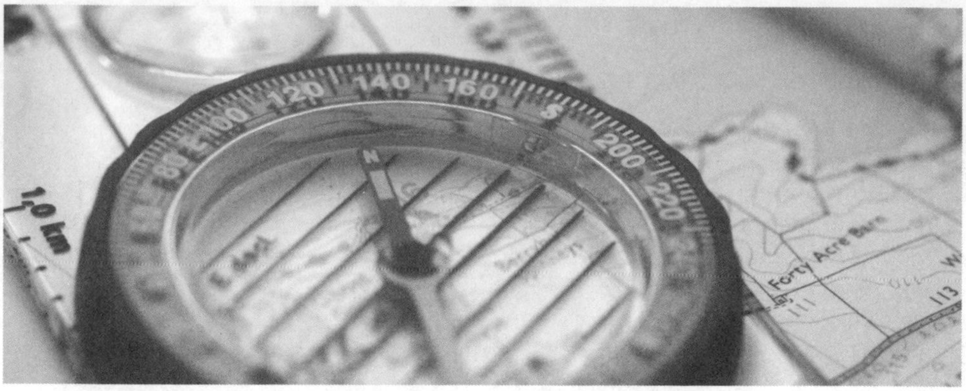

Do Something Unusual!

Optimism is the one quality associated with success and happiness more than any other.

—Brian Tracy

Marketing presented in creative and unusual ways makes an impression on people. Laughter is the greatest stress relief in the world, and people love a good laugh. Do something crazy!

A Few Ideas

Rent a Big Bird or other silly costume, and pay a teenager to stay out in front of your office wearing it and waving people in for an open house. Use your "Silly Holiday" marketing calendar for ideas; for instance, on President's Day, you could have someone outside dressed like George Washington.

Pick an unusual occupation, and announce in your newsletter that you will give a $10 discount to anyone who comes in during that month who can prove they make their living that way. Pick unusual occupations like cemetery plot sales, people who deliver port-a-johns, bee-keepers, or whatever strikes your fancy.

In the summertime, have a lemonade stand outside your office. Kids (under the watchful eye of an adult, of course) can pass out your business cards and discount coupons to everyone who buys a cup.

Most towns that have a small airport usually have someone who gives flying lessons or local pilots who take people on joyrides and sight-seeing tours. Invest in a big banner, and barter massage with the pilot if he'll fly your banner when he's making local flights.

During the holidays, announce that your office is a drop-off place for gifts for the needy. Offer a discount to anyone who brings in an unwrapped new toy or a bag of non-perishable food items. Give the haul to the Salvation Army or other charitable distribution organization.

Many musicians will perform at the drop of a hat. Trade massage with someone who plays an unusual instrument to stand outside your office and play for a couple of hours. A bagpiper in full Scottish regalia would be great! Be out there beside him armed with business cards and brochures. A juggler or bubble blowers (the big bubbles you can stand up in) are other possibilities.

Do you massage pets? Hold a day of doing dog massage—outdoors, in the summertime; you don't want to risk getting any fleas in your office. Advertise a day of dog massage to raise money for the Humane Society. Give the dogs a five or ten-minute massage for a donation and give the owner a discount coupon toward their first massage.

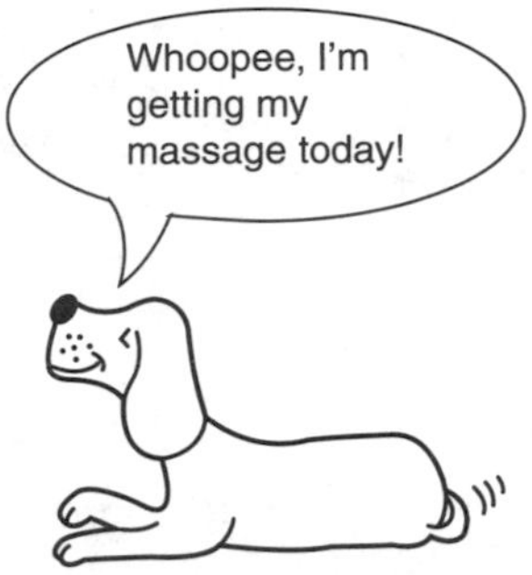

Remember, if it's a charity event, you can get free public service announcements (not to mention spreading good will) for it.

Dress up and decorate the outside of your office on Halloween, and while you're giving out treats to the kids—who in this day and age don't usually go out alone—give the parents a discount coupon for their first massage.

There are a lot of promotional stunts you could do to involve children. Remember, kids have parents—your targeted market—and people are always looking for free and fun events to take their kids to. If you have the space in your parking lot, you could collaborate with local law enforcement by holding a day for kids to be fingerprinted (it's unfortunate that this is a common practice that's become necessary in some places). You can give away something cheap like balloons or rubber balls. Many towns now have a business that specializes in kid's parties with plastic ball houses, inflatable castles, and so forth. You could approach that company and see if they would set up for free in your parking lot—generating publicity for their company and giving out their own business cards—in exchange for helping with your event. Avoid having clowns. A lot of younger kids are scared of clowns; I have witnessed this over and over at events I have participated in. These are just a few ideas. You can probably come up with something just as creative on your own.

Buzz's Story

I really got lucky when I started using the suggestion to offer a discount to people in funny occupations. When I announced in my newsletter what I was doing, a client of mine who is a radio announcer got a wacky idea for a promotion of his own, interviewing people in these weird occupations on the air. He'll announce that the weird occupation this week is ________ and say that the first one to call in who works in that occupation will win a free massage. It's hysterical, and people love it. He does it every Friday morning during drive time on the radio, and the interviewee gets a gift certificate for a free massage—which I am getting radio ads in exchange for.

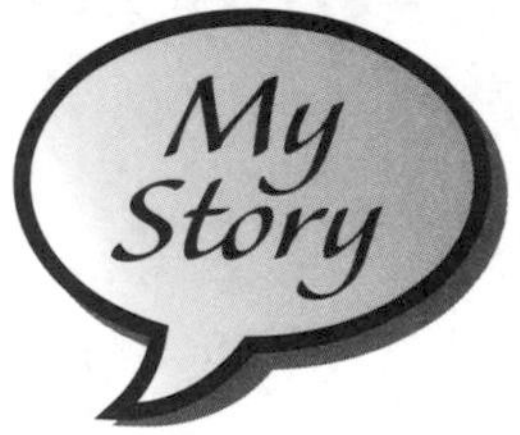

My Personal Journey

This Week's Activity: Do Something Unusual! Date____________________

For this week's activity, you are going to do something unusual to get publicity for your business. Use one of the ideas I've mentioned, or think up your own.

My Goals

____

____

____

What's in my way?

____

____

____

What action can I take to remedy the situation?

____

____

____

One-Year Progress Update Date ____________________

____

____

____

POSITIVE AFFIRMATION: **I have fun while generating publicity and creating abundance for my business.**

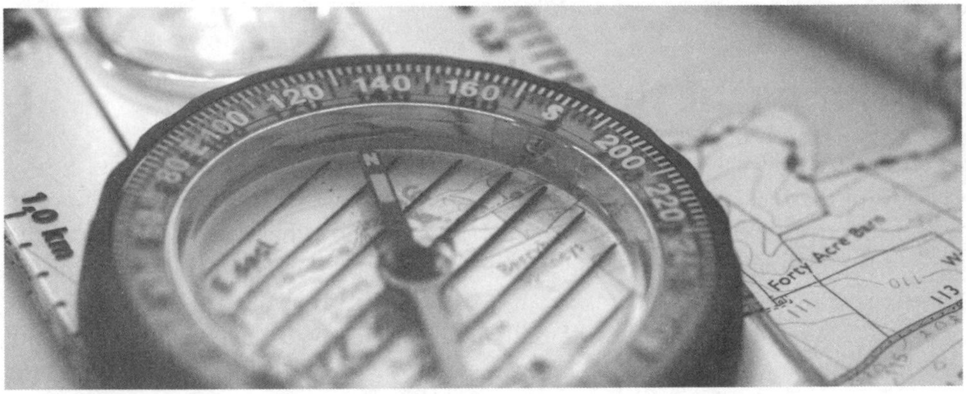

CHAPTER

39

Share Your Space

Success is a process, a quality of mind and a way of being, an outgoing affirmation of life.

—Alex Noble

If you have your own business and own space, even if that's only one room, consider sharing it with another or other practitioners. You're paying for the space; even if you own it clear you're still paying utilities, taxes, insurance, and so forth, and you might as well get the maximum use out of it. Unless you're there 24/7, there are opportunities to share with someone and increase your profits. On the other side, if you are a new therapist who can't afford an office of your own, but still want to be self-employed, you could approach other therapists about sharing their space.

Special Services

When I opened my business, I knew of people here in my town who were traveling somewhere out of town to get services that weren't available here. Although there are a number of massage therapists here, especially due to the presence of a nearby massage school, there were still specialty areas that were lacking.

The end result is that I made arrangements with out-of-town practitioners to travel here, and advertised their presence. On Wednesday, a practitioner comes in to do lymphatic drainage. On Thursdays, a Rolfer comes in. On Fridays, it's the acupuncturist. All of them happen to be traveling from the closest big city, a little over an hour away, and they're all booked up. As I am writing this, the lymphatic drainage specialist has all her appointments filled for the next four months and is not taking any new clients.

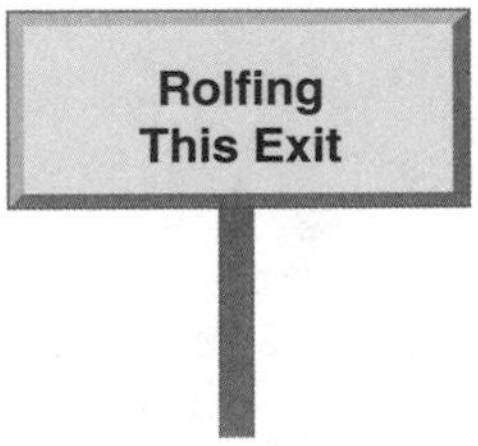

Other than filling specialty niches, another tactic is just filling the hours. If you don't want to work evening hours or weekends, someone else does. A therapist in my office attends worship on Saturday and works on Sunday, and she's always very busy. This a day off for a lot of people, and maybe the only time they have to get a massage. If you take a day off, you're not making any income, and why shouldn't you? Passive income is the very best kind!

Working Out the Details

There are several ways to handle this situation. You can ask for flat rent or a percentage of the fees collected. Whichever way you decide to go, it is best to have a written contract in order to avoid misunderstandings on either side—and stick to the agreement. You may choose to have the agreement renewable yearly, or month by month, if you have any concerns about it working out for you. You may also want to agree on whether or not you will mutually refer clients to each other, whether the practitioner wants you to do bookings for them (or not), what day and how the rent is going to be paid, whether or not they have the use of your linens, phone, and office equipment, what cleaning up after themselves and laundry you would expect them to do, and so forth. The practitioner is going to act as an independent contractor, unless you want to hire an employee.

In either case, if it is agreeable to both parties, you can then market the fact that you have extended hours to accommodate evening appointments, or that you are now open on Saturday and Sunday, or whatever the situation dictates. Extended hours are a great thing for your business—especially if you don't have to work them all yourself. Many people can't take off work during the day to get a massage and will be very glad to know they can get one in the evening, or on Sunday afternoon.

Again, if it's agreeable to both parties, this is another marketing opportunity. It might even be a press release and a photo opportunity—*"Harmony Bodyworks is happy to announce the association of Bill Jones, Certified Rolfer. Bill is a graduate of the Rolf Institute and Gardner-Webb University with a degree in exercise physiology. Bill will be available for appointments every evening between 5 and 9 pm Monday-Friday. Bill resides in the Charlottetown community. We welcome him to our staff."*

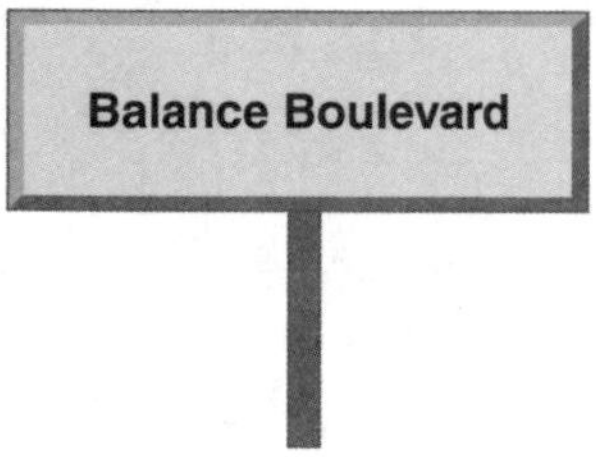

If advertising is to be done, that should also be settled in the contract—who pays for what, who provides linens and oil, and so forth. If everything is addressed up front, there is less chance of conflict later, and more chance for the venture to be successful for everyone involved.

By sharing your space, you will be increasing your own wealth, as well as helping someone else who possibly can't afford their own office, and offering increased benefits to clients.

Student Interns

Another possibility is to have a massage student intern in your space. The fact that they need practice hours can be of great benefit to you and to your clientele as well. Be sure you investigate the law in your state before any money changes hands. In my state, students are not allowed to receive *any* compensation, including tips. The average among the massage schools here is that students have to do between 75 and 150 hours of practice massage for free. Although the student is not allowed to receive money, the therapists or businesses that are sponsoring them may charge a fee for student services. In my area, this is a very common practice in the massage schools, their clinics, and the businesses that have agreed to act as intern venues for students. Again, be sure you operate within the laws governing student massage in your state.

Student massage could be offered at a much reduced rate. If you have clients you know need the work and can't afford it often enough, call and make the offer to them that they can get massage from the student intern in your office for $10, $20, or give it to them free if you feel led to.

The student benefits, because he's getting the practice he needs. Your clients benefit, because they are able to get massage free or at a reduced rate. You benefit, because you are not personally doing the massage, but still getting income from it.

Your clients are getting the perception that you are a benevolent person who enjoys helping people by providing them with this service. The final benefit, of course, is that the student will also massage *you* at no charge. It's a "win-win" situation.

Sunshine's Story

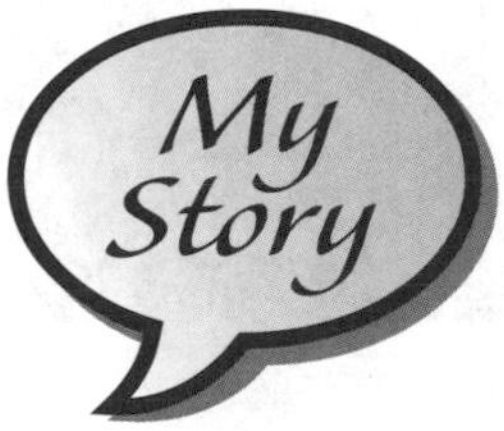

I have school-age children, and I really only want to work while they're in school, but I live too far off the beaten path to have a home practice, so I rent a one-room office in town. I found someone to share my space by sending a notice to the nearest massage school. I got a recent graduate who's a night owl to share the rent and utilities. He comes in as I'm leaving, and it works out great for both of us.

My Personal Journey

This Week's Activity: Sharing Space

Date____________________

For this week's activity, you are going to investigate sharing your space. If you *need* space to share, investigate the possibilities by approaching existing therapy offices that may be willing to share with you. If you *have* space to share, write down a description of what type of therapist you'd be willing to share with, the days and hours the office would be available, the financial and other arrangements you would like to have with that practitioner, and so forth. Consider placing a Classified Ad, or call the other therapists in your town and let them know what you're looking for. If you're looking for specialty practices that don't exist in your town, do an Internet search in the city closest to you and look for someone who would be willing to travel to your office.

My Goals

What's in my way?

What action can I take to remedy the situation?

One-Year Progress Update

Date____________________

POSITIVE AFFIRMATION: **Sharing space benefits me, the therapists I share with, and our clients.**

CHAPTER

40

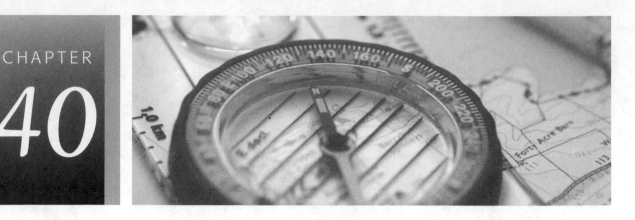

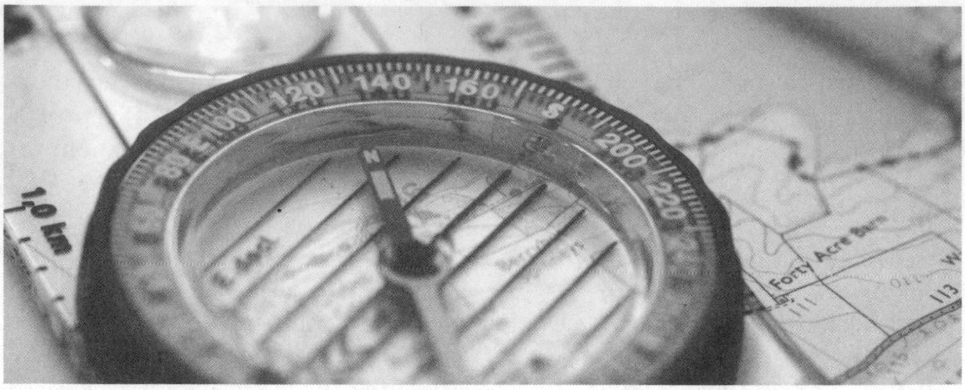

The Power of the Handwritten Note

Self-trust is the first secret of success, the belief that if you are here the authorities of the universe put you here, and for cause, or with some task strictly appointed you in your constitution, and so long as you work at that you are well and successful.

—Ralph Waldo Emerson

In this age of computers, we hardly ever have to write a word with a pen anymore unless we desire to, except our signature—and even that can be stamped or digitally signed. It's time to revive that Victorian pasttime, the handwritten note.

Tropicana Massage
4th St. Arcade at the Beach
Palmfruit, FL 99876
898-444-5555

January 9, 2007

Dear Mrs. McGillicuddy,

Thank you so much for visiting Tropicana Massage earlier this week. In appreciation for your business, here's $10 off your next massage if booked within the next thirty days.

Kitty Mangram, LMT

A Personal Touch

Taking the time to write a handwritten note is a gesture that the recipient will notice, more so than the preprinted postcard, the fancy imprinted Christmas card, and so forth. Even if it's as simple as a thank-you card for a referral, people appreciate the time and thought that goes into a handwritten note. It's a personal touch that says "You're worth the extra time." You should never fail to send a note to doctors and other practitioners who refer to you. It's professional courtesy.

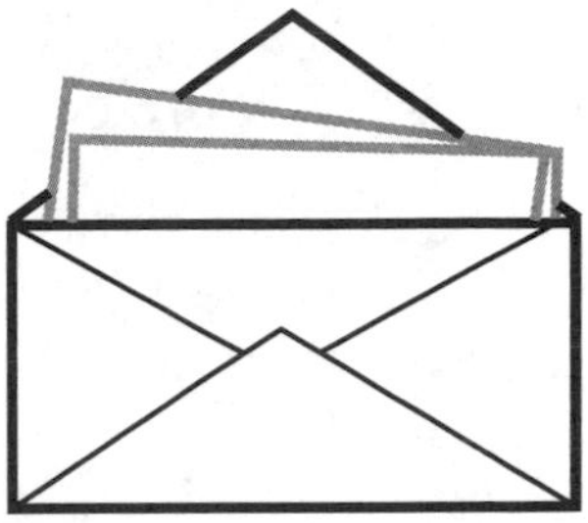

Birthdays, new babies, weddings, congratulatory notes, graduations, sympathy, thank you, are just a few of the opportunities to write a handwritten note. Nice blank note cards can serve the purpose for any occasion. Even if you have preprinted cards, a handwritten note added to them can make a good impression. For instance, you can use the preprinted, "Welcome to my practice" cards, but take the time to write, "Thank you so much for patronizing my business. I appreciate your support." That takes all of two minutes, but the good impression will last longer. Don't worry if your handwriting isn't the greatest; just take your time, be neat, and as long as it's legible, it's fine. You can always print if you have to. It's the thought and the time that went into it that counts.

Especially in small communities, the local newspaper is a gold mine of information about locals—birth announcements, retirements, engagements, marriages, deaths, and so forth, and also human interest stories and news. If one of your clients gets promoted, wins an award, or some other newsworthy happening, send them a "Congratulations on your new job and best wishes for your success" or something similar. If you don't know what to say, most card and graphics software programs have templates with appropriate sayings, etiquette books cover the subject, and the Internet has whole websites devoted to "what to say in any situation." For a sympathy note, keep it simple like, "I'm so sorry for the loss of your brother." Flowery words aren't necessary. It's the thought that counts, and sending a handwritten note lets the client know that you have taken an extra minute to think about them. Word of mouth is the best advertising, and personal touches will make people talk favorably about you just as much, if not more, than your technical expertise.

Don't forget about clients you haven't seen in a long time, either. A handwritten note might bring them back to the fold: "Dear Mrs. Smith, I haven't heard from you lately. I hope your absence means your TMJ hasn't bothered you since your last session. Please give me a call when I can be of service." Enclose a business card and a brochure. Maybe they've just been busy and haven't thought of you in a while, and a handwritten note serves that purpose—to make them think about you.

Paige's Story

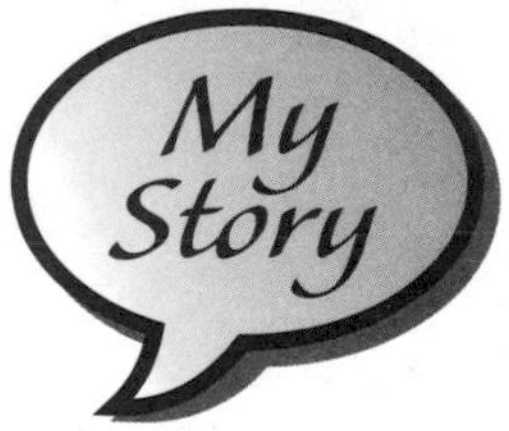

Every new client receives a handwritten "thank you for your business" card within a day or two of their visit. If they didn't rebook at the time of their first visit, I also include a coupon for $10 off their next massage if it's within the next 30 days. It gets quite a few people who wouldn't reschedule on the spot to get back in sooner rather than later.

My Personal Journey

This Week's Activity: Sending Handwritten Notes Date____________________

For this week's activity, you are going to write handwritten notes. If you're still a student, try preparing handwritten notes to those people you have given student massages to, thanking them for allowing you to practice on them, reminding them that you'll soon be licensed, and hope you'll see them soon in your new practice. If you're in practice, look through your files and make sure you've thanked people for referrals. Get in the habit of checking the newspaper for clients who have done something newsworthy, gotten married recently, or experienced some other event that would be a suitable occasion for sending a handwritten note. Then send them!

My Goals

____

____

____

What's in my way?

____

____

____

What action can I take to remedy the situation?

____

____

____

One-Year Progress Update Date____________________

____

____

____

POSITIVE AFFIRMATION: **My handwritten notes make people feel special.**

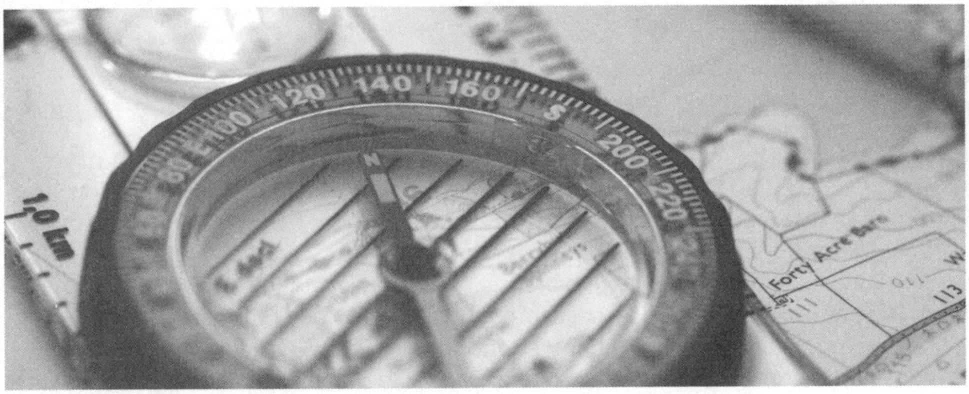

CHAPTER 41

Massage Parties

The best augury of a man's success in his profession is that he thinks it is the finest in the world.

—George Eliot

Massage parties are a fun way to meet new potential clients and to introduce them to your services. A massage party works on the same principle as other home product parties (*remember, you are the product*). You need someone who is willing to host the party in their home and who has some friends to invite over for a couple of hours. You can provide the host with nice invitations with your business imprint on them. An ideal number of attendees for a two-hour party is around 8 to 12 guests. You should gift the hostess with a free massage for hosting.

You're Invited to a Massage Party!

When: Sunday, January 15, 4:00–6:00 pm
Where: The Home of Lucille Rollins
444 Bennett Rd., Gilkey NC

Massage provided by
Carla Trainum, LMBT

rsvp 828-288-3727

I'm going to stop right here to state that I am not talking about a Cuddle Party. If you haven't yet heard of Cuddle Parties, information about them is all over the Internet. They have grown so popular that in February of 2007, AMTA felt compelled to address the issue through the following press release posted on their website (www.amtamassage.org):

AMTA Not Associated with Cuddle Party Programs

Evanston, IL – The American Massage Therapy Association (AMTA) does not have and never has had any connection with Cuddle Parties. Neither the association nor its chapters accept participation in a Cuddle Party, or training as a facilitator toward Continuing Education requirements.

Regrettably, an AMTA chapter volunteer mistakenly announced that participation in these parties is accepted toward massage Continuing Education requirements, and the AMTA chapter announced it is able to approve hours of continuing education for it. The National Certification Board for Therapeutic Massage and Bodywork (NCBTMB) approves providers of massage Continuing Education. AMTA and most of its chapters are approved by NCBTMB as providers. However, neither AMTA nor its chapters can approve providers of training programs. Also, AMTA does not endorse products or services, and does not promote or endorse activities that are not massage.

AMTA regrets that this misinformation about the association has been circulated and that it has misled massage therapists, the Cuddle Party organization and the public.

Cuddle Parties, according to the founders, are all about boundary-appropriate, safe, nonsexual touching, including massage and other exercises in touching other human beings. It has been rumored that massage therapists could get Continuing Education credit for attending and/or facilitating Cuddle Parties. According to the above statement from AMTA, and the listing of approved classes on the NCBTMB website (www.ncbtmb.com), this is not true. As a professional massage therapist, you must be very diligent in your mission to avoid any appearance of sexual impropriety. Cuddle Parties may be harmless and even therapeutic, but the potential is there for misunderstanding of your intent if you were to host such a thing, just by the very name of it. Leave it for someone else.

At the beginning of your massage party, introduce yourself, talk about where your business is located, your menu of services, your prices and hours of operation, the benefits of massage, the package deals you offer, and so forth. This part of the party should last around a half hour. Be sure to ask if there are any questions. Have plenty of brochures and your business cards on hand—and bring along your appointment book and a supply of gift certificates as well. If you have promo items, such as pens or sticky notes, give everybody one. Set your massage chair or table up in an out-of-the-way place, and give the attendees free ten-minute massages while everyone is eating and visiting.

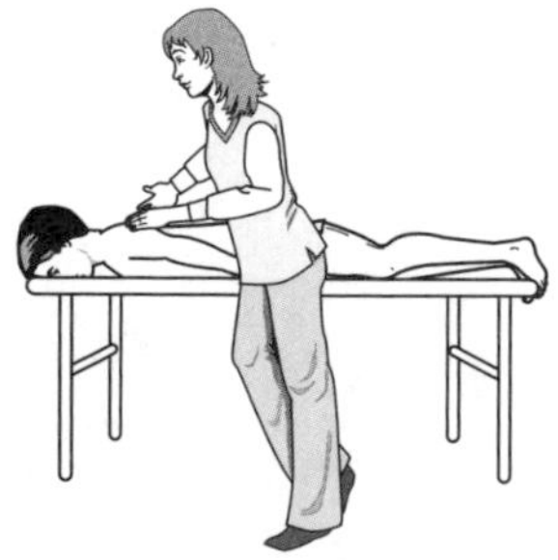

Announce that anyone who purchases a gift certificate or books a massage at the party will receive a discount for booking right then. Also announce that anyone can earn a free massage by hosting a party in *their* home—and it's wise to stipulate that at least six of the guests should be people who aren't present at this one. The objective is to keep being introduced to new people who are potential clients.

These parties are particularly lucrative when you hold them a short while prior to holidays—Christmas, Mother's Day, and Valentine's Day—when people can conveniently do all their shopping while they're sitting right there.

My Story

Joli's Story

The first time I did massage at a bridal shower, I got two other bookings from it, and it snowballed from there. I usually do a shower or bridal party at least twice a month, and it's all been by word-of-mouth advertising.

Another possibility is to be available to do massage at parties that aren't necessarily massage parties. Choose carefully; parties where the clients are drinking or all members of the opposite sex are not a good idea. Bridal parties are great; family reunions and those type gatherings are a safer bet.

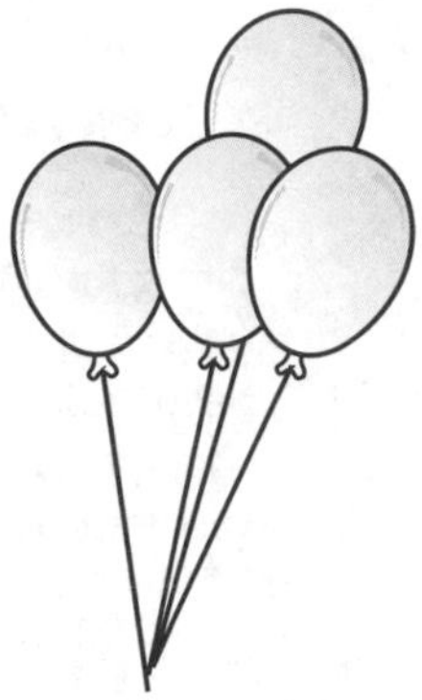

One therapist I know has a client who is a multi-level marketer and very successful. Every month she hosts a big party at her home for her down line; it's half sales meeting and half socializing, and she hires the therapist for the day to give the attendees massage to the tune of $80 an hour plus a nice tip. When the weather's nice, it's a cookout held poolside; other times it's a fancy catered meal, of which the therapist also gets to avail herself. In addition to the money, the lovely surroundings, and the nice meal, she also gets to hand out her business cards and brochures, and always takes her appointment book and gift certificates along. It's a fun and lucrative day.

One caveat: people love to receive free massage. If your intent is to serve the poor by giving free massage, that's admirable, so go ahead. But if your intent is to work massage parties with the potential to increase your business and your income, you want to hold these parties in the homes of people who can afford to pay for massage and whose friends and neighbors are people who can afford to pay for massage.

My Personal Journey

This Week's Activity: Marketing with Massage Parties Date____________________

For this week's activity, you are going to increase your business by way of a massage party. Resolve that during the coming year, you are going to do six massage parties (at least). Write that intention down. Type up a short list of directions and details for the person who is going to host the party telling them what they need to do—namely, invite the people (with the invitations you provide), have a place where you can set your massage table or chair up, provide a few snacks, and prepare to have a good visit with friends. Create your invitations. Ask your existing customers if they'd be willing to host one in exchange for a free massage. Put a catchy sign in your office announcing the availability of massage parties. Announce it in your newsletter and in an e-mail blast.

My Goals

____

____

____

What's in my way?

____

____

____

What action can I take to remedy the situation?

____

____

____

One-Year Progress Update Date____________________

____

____

____

POSITIVE AFFIRMATION: **Creating my prosperity is a lot of fun.**

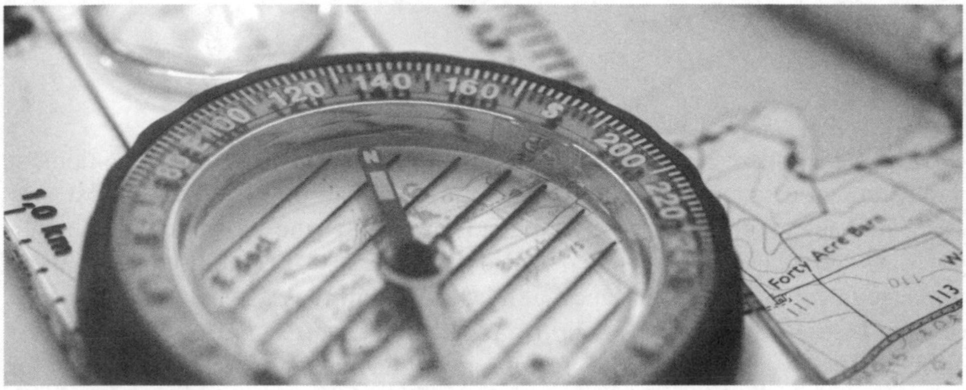

CHAPTER

42

Public Access Television

> *For you to be successful, sacrifices must be made. It's better that they are made by others, but failing that, you'll have to make them yourself.*
>
> —Rita Mae Brown

One of the most exciting media developments in the past century is public access television. In the 1970s, when cable television was still new, the Federal Communications Commission decreed that cable companies in the 100 largest markets in the United States were obligated to provide three channels that were to be used for state and local governments, for education, and for the general public for noncommercial use. Don't let the fact that it's noncommercial deter you from taking advantage of it. In case you're not familiar with it, check your TV guide for the channels and watch your local Public Access channels. They're very diverse—shows about everything from how to maximize your soybean crop to how to do T'ai Chi. Exercise and healthy living shows abound on Public Access television. A show on massage will fit right in.

Sally's Story

My Story

I'm certified in equine massage. There is already a public access show on massage in my area; it airs once a week. I always try to watch it, and I noticed that they had never had a show on equine massage, so I contacted the host and proposed a show on it. They took me up on it, and they filmed me doing a massage on a horse, which led to my getting invited to appear on another show about horses. It was a great experience and I got a lot of mileage out of it, publicity-wise, and got some new clients out of it too. People called me because they had seen me on television. And like other television shows, it's on every now and then as a rerun—just a bonus.

It's Free

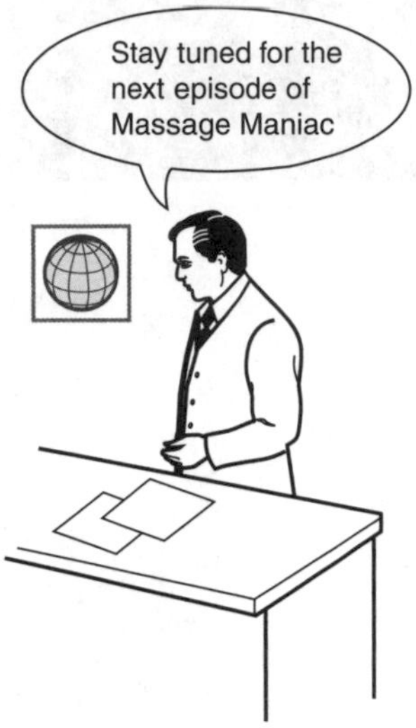
Stay tuned for the next episode of Massage Maniac

Most cable companies provide free air time, free facilities, free use of equipment and technical personnel (they're obligated to), making it possible for almost anyone who has the time and desire to do their own television show. So even though you can't do a blatant commercial for your business, you could do a show about massage in general, or, for instance, a show about how massage helps specific conditions. Doesn't that open the door to a long-running series in itself? Massage for carpal tunnel syndrome, massage for fibromyalgia, massage for TMJ, massage for injury recovery, massage for pregnant women, and the list is as long as there are conditions—and *you're the star*. There are so many different modalities of massage and bodywork now, if you highlighted one a week, you'd be on the air for years to come.

The Domino Effect

Having a public access television show is certainly newsworthy. Visualize the story in your local paper: "Heather Wiltse, local massage therapist who owns The Body in Balance in Ruffton, will be appearing in a new show called *Massage for Everyone* on Public Access channel 35 on the Northstar Cable System. Wiltse has been practicing massage for ten years, and each week will be highlighting a different condition that massage can help. She plans to have local physicians, chiropractors, clients who have been helped by massage, and other practitioners as guests on the show. Tune in each Tuesday at 10 a.m. following the farm report."

You might get a radio interview out of it, too. Put it in your newsletter. Send an announcement to your e-mail list. Hang a big sign in your office. Rent a flashing sign and put it outside your office. Getting your own television show is a big event! And even though it isn't technically a commercial for your business, there's no doubt that it'll get your name out to the public. Appearing on the Public Access channel might even get you invited onto another local station to talk about your show. It's the "domino effect."

You might think this is too grandiose a plan—you're not an actor, or a writer. You don't have to be! If you have an idea for a show (feel free to use the one above), approach your local cable company. Call and ask for an appointment with the person in charge of public access. They'll tell you exactly what you need to know, such as whether you have to have a written script prepared, do they get to approve it, what color clothing to wear to show up best, what you have to personally do and how to do it, and what they will be doing for you.

And on the off-chance that there is already a show about massage on Public Access in your area, call the host and pitch them the possibility of having you on the show. For that matter, call your local commercial station and ask *them* to have you on the show; they do a segment on human interest or a personal or business story every day, and it might as well be about you. If you don't ask, you'll never know.

My Personal Journey

This Week's Activity: Getting a Television Appearance Date____________

For this week's activity, you are going try to get a television appearance. If you're still a student, plan ahead for doing this activity when you get licensed. Call your local cable company and make an appointment to see the person in charge of Public Access programming. You're just gathering information. Find out the terms and requirements of getting a show on the air, how long the process takes, how often the show could run. Be sure you have written down a list of questions to ask so you won't forget anything. After you have time to consider all the factors involved and decided you can commit the time and effort it will take, call the programmer for another appointment and pitch your show. *Hollywood, here you come*!

My Goals

What's in my way?

What action can I take to remedy the situation?

One-Year Progress Update Date____________

POSITIVE AFFIRMATION: **I am worthy of receiving attention and financial gain.**

CHAPTER 43

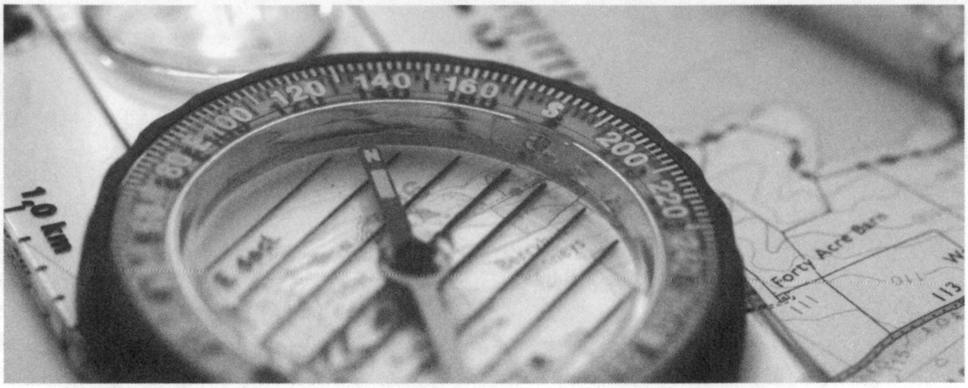

Monday Morning Schedule Blitz

If you wish success in life, make perseverance your bosom friend, experience your wise counselor, caution your elder brother and hope your guardian genius.

—Joseph Addison

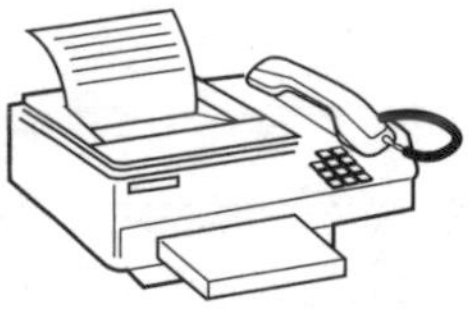

Wouldn't it be great to look at your appointment book on Monday morning and see it filled for the whole week? Then try this: when you get to work on Monday morning, make a list of the appointment times you have available. Then e-mail and/or broadcast fax a short note to your client list:

> Dear Clients of Bayside Massage & Bodywork,
>
> The following appointment times are available at our office for the coming week:
>
> ______________________________
>
> Please call to schedule an appointment today—you'll be glad you did! 288-8888
> Your Massage Therapist,
>
> Susie Marks, LMT

That's all there is to it. The phone is going to ring within a few minutes of doing this. Believe it!

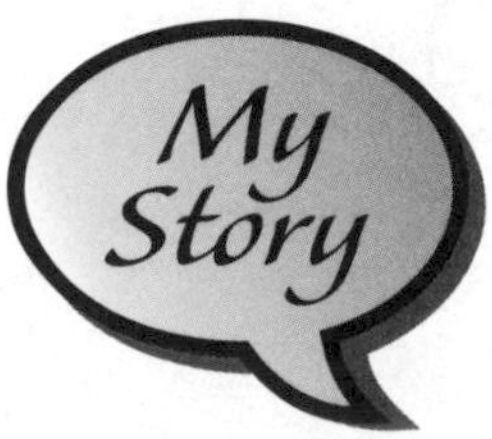

Terence's Story

I read about the Monday morning schedule blitz on a marketing website a couple of years ago and did it the very next Monday. I wondered it if would work—and I didn't have to wonder long. The phone started ringing! It has the effect of spurring those people who are procrastinating to make an appointment before their chosen time gets given away. I've done it every week since. It works!

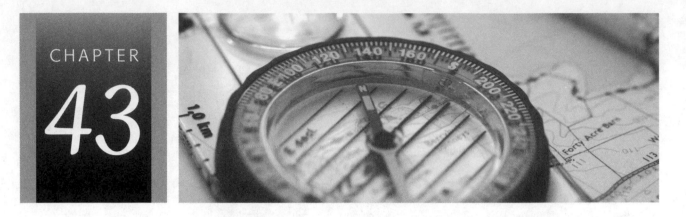

My Personal Journey

This Week's Activity: Monday Morning Schedule Blitz

Date________________________

For this week's activity, you are going to do the Monday Morning Schedule Blitz. If you are still a student who lacks practice hours, you can do it too. Compose your message, send it out, and believe that you are going to fill those appointments. Make it a habit to do this every single week.

My Goals

____

____

____

What's in my way?

____

____

____

What action can I take to remedy the situation?

____

____

____

One-Year Progress Update

Date________________________

____

____

____

POSITIVE AFFIRMATION: **My appointment book is filled with abundance.**

CHAPTER

44

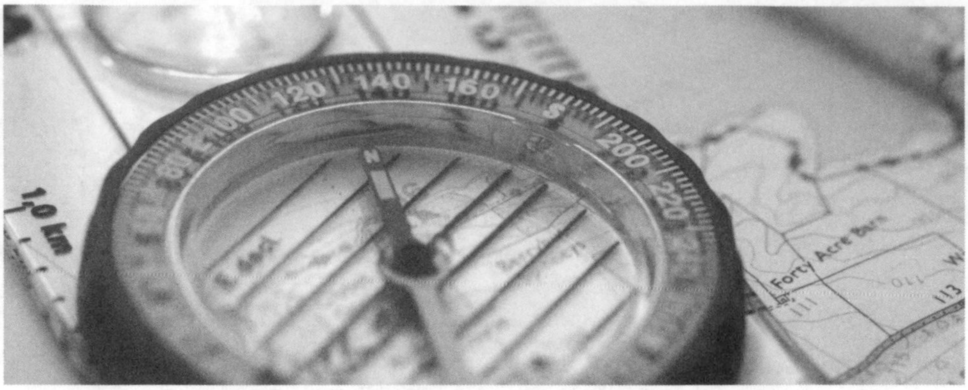

Advertising in Unusual Places

If your success is not on your own terms, if it looks good to the world but does not feel good in your heart; it is not success at all.

—Anna Quindlen

The bottom line for deciding where to put your advertising dollars is how much it costs divided by how many people are going to see it. Chapter 3 was a discussion of venues that are often a waste of money because of the limited number of people who will see it. When it comes to *any* choice in spending for advertising, always do the math—and sometimes, you're going to consider a few other factors—as mentioned in the same chapter—if it's your 8-year-old son asking you to buy an ad on the little league calendar, of course you're going to do it. For advertising opportunities that have a limited audience, other than your son's ball team, consider the price. If it's only going to reach 500 people and it cost $100, pass it by, but if they're selling ads for $10, that's not a bad deal.

Another thing to consider is whether or not the person who is approaching you to buy limited-exposure ad space is a supporter of *your* business. While you might not be excited about advertising on restaurant menus, if the person who owns the restaurant happened to be a good client of yours who has referred a lot of people to you, you would and should probably do it. It's a benefit to the community when small businesses support each other.

Places to Place Your Ad

There are a lot of opportunities to advertise in odd places. It seems like everything these days except the air we breathe is subsidized by advertising. Here are some opportunities you may not have thought about as places for an ad:

- Grocery carts
- Bus-stop benches
- Bowling alley or golf course scorecards
- On paper cups (donate those to the concession stand at your son's ball team instead of buying an ad on the calendar)
- On a stock car at the local race track (we're not talking NASCAR, unless you're already so successful you don't need to be reading this book)

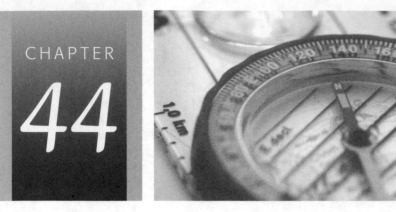

- Phone booths
- Book marks—donate them to local libraries and used bookstores
- In a kiosk at the airport
- On coffee cups in a busy restaurant

In addition to placing ads, be creative with the places you leave your business cards, brochures, and flyers. Flyers printed on neon-colored paper in bold black print are eye-catching. Always have some in your car and put one on every bulletin board you encounter; after all, they're *free*. If there's a local college campus, go systematically through the buildings and put one on every bulletin board. Health food stores, hospitals, community centers, service stations, town squares, city hall, the local tourism office, golf courses, recreation centers, gyms, local parks, and anywhere else you see a board—seize the opportunity to put up an eye-catching flyer. Printing them so there are tear-offs on the bottom with your business name and phone number is a great idea.

Danita's Story

It's amazing how many bulletin boards you can find around town, and I have made it my business to put my flyers on every one I can find. I always ask new clients how they heard about my business and half the time the answer is they saw my flyer on a bulletin board.

The Billboard Alternative

Billboards are expensive and out of the range of many of us, especially those just starting out in business. Ask your grandparents or anyone old enough to have been around in the 1930's through the 1950's about Burma Shave signs. I think that's a great form of advertising that ought to be resurrected. They're fun!

Burma Shave was a shaving lotion, made by a small family concern and the sales weren't taking off. In 1925, the owner of the company's son got an idea for these signs, and even though his father thought it was a waste of money, he agreed to give his son $200 to get the signs made. And of course in 1925, $200 was a small fortune. He ended up putting more than 7000 signs all across America and their business was soaring. We're not talking about across America here—just a half-mile or so stretch of the road on the way to the office.

Burma Shave signs were small wooden signs, red with white lettering, always in poetic form, usually quite humorous, and usually grouped in groups of five or six signs along a stretch of highway so people read them in sequence. People loved reading them. Here's a sample, adapted for a massage business named *Massage Corps*:

Table 44.1 Burma Shave-type Signs

Feeling stressed	Aching head	Tension here	Got stress?	One more block
Achy and sore	Hurting feet	Tension there	In a mess?	Almost here
Don't have to Feel that way no more	Feeling like you've been beat?	Tension, tension everywhere?	We can help you feel your best	You'll feel the best you've felt in years
Massage Corps	Massage Corps	Massage Corps	Massage Corps	Massage Corps

A local barbecue restaurant in my town has adopted signs like these and the owner has told me they get a lot of comments on them—always positive—about how people enjoy reading them. The signs are small so they're low-cost. You just have to do a little legwork to get permission to place them, either from your state's Department of Transportation or the property owners themselves. Be sure to follow your local laws governing signage.

My Personal Journey

This Week's Activity: Advertise in Unusual Places Date____________

For this week's activity, you are going to find some unusual places to advertise in—and do it! Start by making flyers and take them to at least a dozen places around town that have bulletin boards. Keep a list of your locations and check back on them frequently to replace them.

My Goals

___

___

___

What's in my way?

___

___

___

What action can I take to remedy the situation?

___

___

___

One-Year Progress Update Date____________

___

___

___

POSITIVE AFFIRMATION: **My advertisements attract attention wherever they are.**

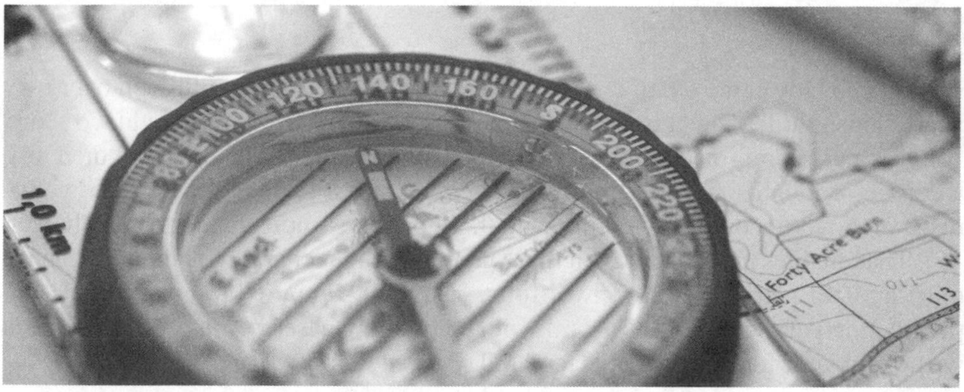

CHAPTER

45

Conducting Research Projects

I learned this, at least, by my experiment; that if one advances confidently in the direction of his dreams, and endeavors to live the life which he has imagined, he will meet with a success unexpected in common hours.

—Henry David Thoreau

Whether you are a new graduate or a therapist with many years experience, consider conducting research in the field of massage and bodywork. This serves multiple purposes and can have multiple benefits. 1) You can gain new clients; 2) you can gain new knowledge, or reinforce a theory you have had; 3) you can document your findings and submit them for publication to one of the massage therapy journals, or even a book publisher; 4) you can gain other media attention from the effort, such as an article in the human interest section of the newspaper, if one of your subjects will agree to speak out.

Getting Clients to Participate

Classified ads are normally very cheap to place in comparison with display ads, and people do read them. Place an ad under "Announcements" advertising that you are conducting research on the effect of massage therapy on ______ (condition), and that participants will receive massage at a reduced rate for agreeing to participate (or you may want to do it gratis if you can afford to). Choose a condition that fascinates you.

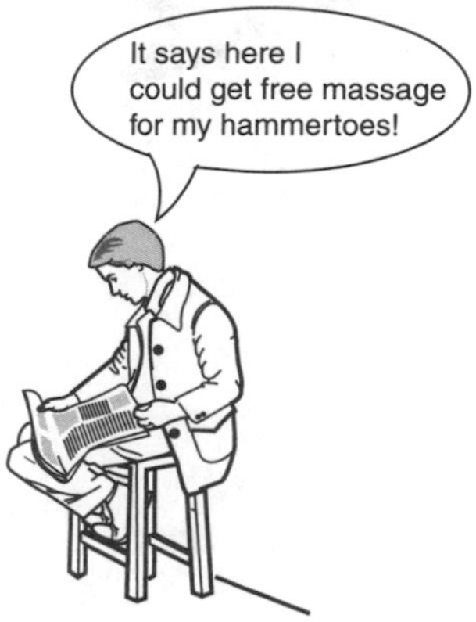
It says here I could get free massage for my hammertoes!

When you get participants—and shoot for several, although you don't necessarily have to have them all at the same time—ask them to sign a release form stating that they acknowledge that you are conducting scientific research and that though their name will be changed to protect their privacy, that they do give permission for details of their case and treatment to be published. Of course, if any of them agree to give testimonials after the fact, that is another benefit to you.

A few years ago, I received a call from a family member who wanted me to work on her mother, who was in a persistent vegetative state following a severe stroke. The lady came out of the condition and spoke for the first time in over two years. This gratified and fascinated me so that I found other cases I could work on. Another person returned to the world of the living, while yet another one died just a couple of months after I started working with him. I applied for and received a research grant to continue working with these patients (more about that in Chapter 46). That enables me to work with these people without charging them any money, but I am still getting paid for my efforts. I haven't submitted to any journals for publication yet; I would like to work with a few more cases before I do, but I have written about it for our state chapter AMTA newsletter.

Fringe Benefits

Another interesting opportunity came my way when a mother called me about her 15-year-old daughter who has Tourette syndrome. The teenager had been under the care of a psychiatrist for the stress she was under due to her diagnosis (Tourette is a neurological condition, not a psychiatric one). The psychiatrist, an older male, realized that he wasn't connecting with the girl and recommended that she receive massage for her stress. Her mother is a single mother and their finances are tight, but I was fascinated by her case and asked the mother if she could afford to pay $10 a session. I have worked on the young lady weekly for about six months and her symptoms have improved. I have advertised for others with the condition but so far have not gotten any, but I have no doubt they'll come along.

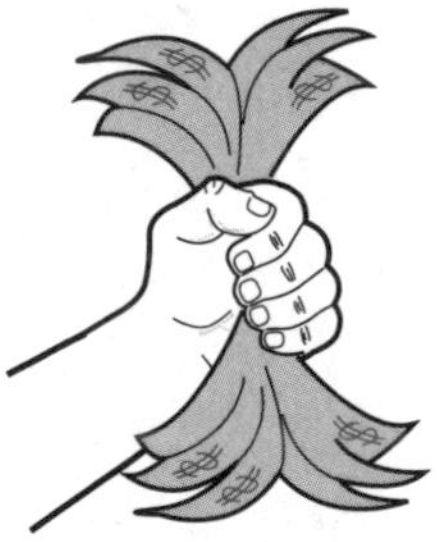

The mother has been very grateful for the massage I have been giving her daughter, and as a thank-you, mobilized her entire family to come and buy gift certificates from my office for Christmas. Her family members came out of the woodwork and in total bought over $800 worth of gift certificates.

You may not be in a financial position to do three or four research clients at a time, so just do one. Do whatever you can do. It will come back to you many times.

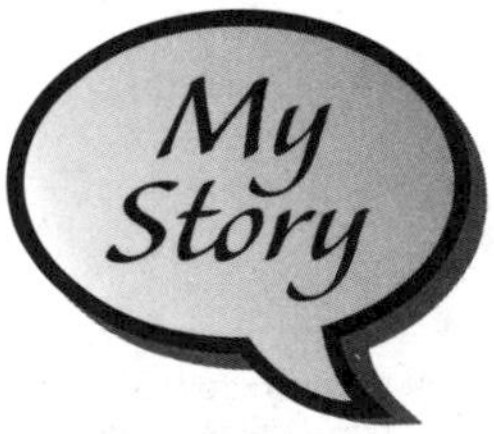

Joyce's Story

I have been collecting research on the effects of massage on people who suffer from an anxiety disorder, because I suffer from it myself. When I first started receiving massage and saw how much it helped me to feel more calm and in balance, I decided to share my story with others. Now it almost seems that I attract people who have the disorder as clients without making any special effort. They view me as a kindred spirit as well as their massage therapist. Someday I'll compile my research along with my personal story into a book.

Documenting Your Findings

A professional massage therapist keeps notes on every massage, usually the universally accepted SOAP notes such as these:

SOAP Notes

S: Stands for *subjective*, or what the client *states*: Lower back hurts, 6 on a scale of 1-10. Particularly painful when sitting in the car.

O: Stands for *objective*, or what the therapist *observed*: taut bands in latissimus dorsi; trigger points around erectors in lumbar area and gluteals.

A: Stands for *action*; what you did with the client: 30 minutes of Swedish massage to get the client loosened up, followed by 20 minutes of neuromuscular therapy and passive stretching to the lumbar area. Client stated pain level at 1-2 after the session.

P: Stands for *plan*; what you would like for the client to do: Suggested a warm bath with Epsom salts and an increase in water intake in order to flush toxins and hydrate the muscle. Suggested that client return for follow-up visit in 3-4 days.

For the purpose of scientific research, you will want to go beyond that. You could ask your clients to fill out self-reports. For instance, prior to the massage, ask them to rate their discomfort or certain symptoms on a scale of 1–10. Then ask them to rate it immediately after the massage, one day later, one week later, and so forth. If it's allowed in the scope of practice in your state, gather scientific information by checking their blood pressure before and after the massage. If you're studying diabetics, you could ask them to check their sugar levels before and after the massage. There are so many possibilities. You may occasionally get a client suffering from a rare condition that's interesting to you, but it won't make a good study if you only have one client. You will need to choose a project that you can at least get a small group of people who have the condition in order to gather enough data to make a valid study. Repetitive motion injuries such as carpal tunnel syndrome, range of motion problems, or chronic conditions like TMJ dysfunction or fibromyalgia make good studies. Set a goal for the study, such as seeing each client for *x* number of visits over a certain time frame, and at the end of that time, compile your data. For good ideas and helpful information, check out the many studies that have been performed by Dr. Tiffany Field and others at the Touch Institute at the University of Miami Medical School. Many of her articles have been published in the trade journals and are also available in the archives on the website at http://www6.miami.edu/touch-research.

If you are conducting research that you hope to publish in a peer-reviewed journal, you need to use scientifically accepted methods of research. Two good sources of information are *Designing Clinical Research* (Hulley, S., et al, 2006, Lippincott Williams & Wilkins) and *Essentials of Research Methods in Health, Physical Education, Exercise Science, and Recreation* (Berg, K. and Latin, R., 2003, Lippincott Williams & Wilkins). You may discover something that helps all mankind. Good luck with your projects!

My Personal Journey

This Week's Activity: Conducting Research Date____________

For this week's activity, you are going to plan a research project on the efficacy of massage. Peruse your client files for people who are suffering from the same condition, or advertise for new clients with a certain condition you'd like to study. Create a standardized form with the measurements or symptoms you want to track, and create a release form for your clients to sign.

My Goals

What's in my way?

What action can I take to remedy the situation?

One-Year Progress Update Date____________

POSITIVE AFFIRMATION: **My research benefits me and my clients.**

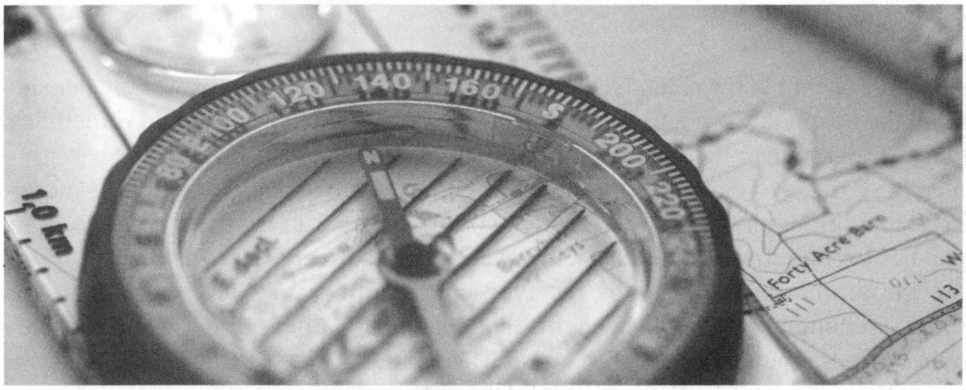

CHAPTER

46

Get a Grant for Doing Massage

People are beginning to see that the first requisite for success in this life is to be a good animal.

—Herbert Spencer

Community service was discussed in Chapter 17, and it's a great thing. Doing research has been discussed in Chapter 45, and that's a great thing also. However, any time that you can perform a needed service for a population that is in need, there is an opportunity to get a grant. Getting a grant allows you the freedom to perform a valuable service to people in need and still get paid for it. Research doesn't have to be part of your grant application, but it may carry more weight with certain entities that give out money than just the benevolent act of doing massage. It depends on whom you approach for money.

Deserving Populations

First, let's look at some populations who could benefit greatly from massage, but perhaps can't afford to get it:

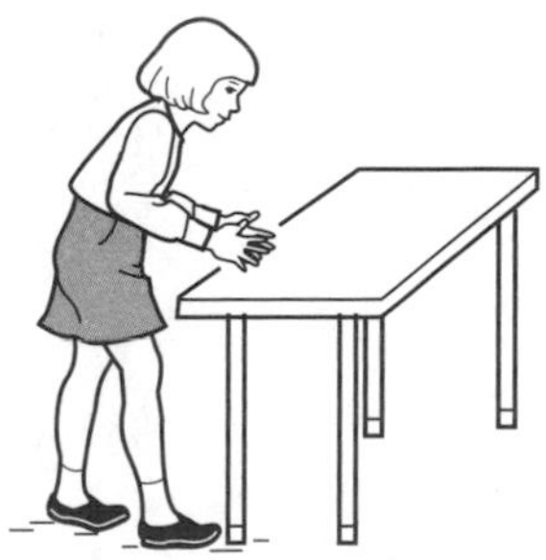

- Residents at an abused women's shelter
- Patients in the VA hospital
- Cancer patients in the oncology ward
- People in homeless shelters
- Crack babies
- Premature babies
- People in nursing homes
- Anyone suffering from any condition that is of personal interest to you and not contraindicated for massage therapy
- Caregivers
- Anyone in need

A therapist I know recently lost a sister to cancer. While she was visiting her sister in the hospital, she got to know some of the other patients, and would sometimes just sit and rub their hands and feet. The doctor came in one day while she was giving a foot rub, and ended up asking her to volunteer on the cancer ward one morning per week, with the promise that he would assist her in trying to get a grant to pay her for her efforts. After just a few weeks, and collaborating with her in filling out the grant application, they received enough money to pay her a half-time salary—enough to get her the benefits that the hospital offers, and she still runs her own business the other half of the week. The patients are so grateful for the massage. The patient's families are grateful. The therapist is grateful to have a certain amount of guaranteed income and health insurance. The doctor and the nurses on the ward are grateful, as her services have made a difference in patient attitudes. It's a win-win situation for everyone.

Where to Get the Money

You don't need a doctor to help you get a grant, but it might be helpful to you to attend a seminar on grant-writing. Many community foundations offer these seminars at no charge a couple of times a year, because believe it or not, they *want* to give away money! It's why they're in business, and many non-profits are in fact obligated to give money away.

Libraries have books on how to obtain grants and information on sources of money. The Internet has plenty of information on corporations and foundations that give grants, and even in some cases applications that you can download on the spot. The American Massage Therapy Association gives annual grants, and some of the other professional associations may as well. Other sources of grants include civic groups, ethnic and religious organizations, private philanthropists, colleges and universities, and many, many more. If you don't ask, you'll never receive!

My Story

Lindsay's Story

I was sexually abused as a child. About the same time I started massage school, I joined a support group for women who were abuse survivors. I shared my dream with the group, which was to use massage to help women who have been abused get used to receiving touch that is positive, nurturing, and non-threatening. The support group uses the anonymity principles of 12-step groups, so even though we share deep, dark secrets, I was very surprised one night after the meeting when a woman came up to me and said her husband was on the board of such-and-such foundation and she bet they would give me a grant. She introduced me to him and they helped me through the whole process of applying. I got the grant money just after I was licensed and it was enough that I could really do a lot of volunteer work at a time I otherwise would have been worrying about getting a business established. It has been a huge blessing to me and the women who have been victimized, too.

My Personal Journey

This Week's Activity: Getting a Grant to Do Massage Date________________

For this week's activity, you are going to research getting a grant to do massage. Go to the library and check out a book on grant writing, or arrange to attend a workshop on the subject. Figure out what population you would like to work with, and do Internet research on possible sources of funding for the grant. If you are still a student, you will likely have to wait until you are licensed before applying for the grant, but you can still go ahead and lay the groundwork. Make a list of sources that you could apply to and practice writing your grant and cover letter. If you're licensed and ready, send it in!

My Goals

___

___

___

What's in my way?

___

___

___

What action can I take to remedy the situation?

___

___

___

One-Year Progress Update Date________________

___

___

___

POSITIVE AFFIRMATION: **The universe wants to share wealth with me so I may share with others.**

CHAPTER 47

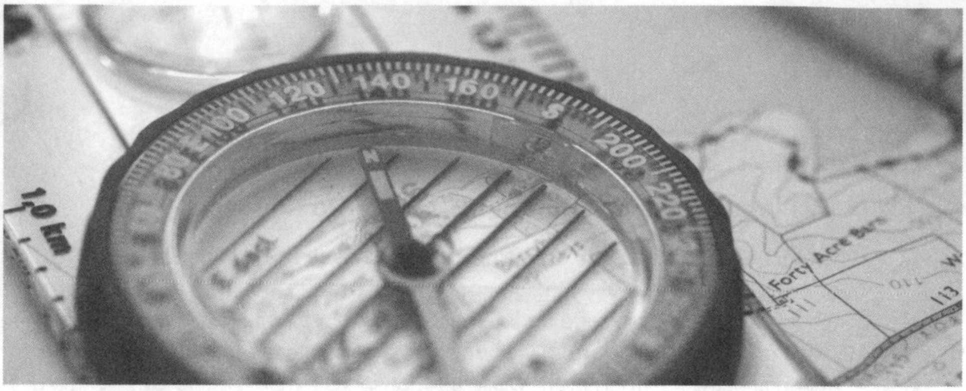

Getting Published

A successful person is one who can lay a firm foundation with the bricks that others throw at him.

—David Brink

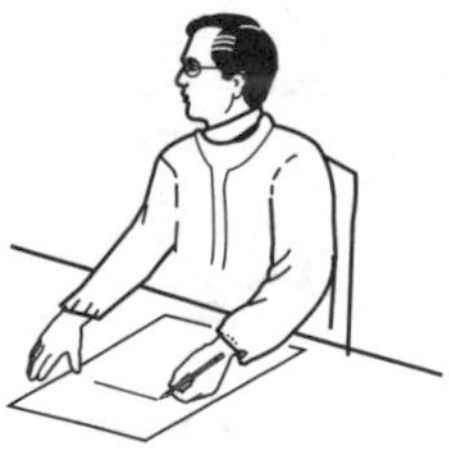

You don't have to be an author or English major to get published. You just have to have an interesting story, something that will engage people's attention, make them laugh—or make them cry, teach them something new, or remind them of something they haven't thought of in a long time.

Think of your experiences during massage school. Weren't some of them emotionally overwhelming, and profoundly enlightening in some way? Looking back at mine, I can recall moments that were hysterically funny, and others that were cathartic; I witnessed myself and others having emotional meltdowns, and growing into something we had never been before, all because of the power of touch. That growth has continued throughout my path today. The human body has a lot to show us, and each day brings something new.

Your Journal

Part of the purpose of this book, as evidenced at the end of each chapter, is to encourage journaling as a way of keeping track of your success. Writing about the day's or the week's events, and revisiting that the next year or five years from now is proof of how far you've come in your journey. Those notes about clients you've helped (anonymously, of course, unless you have a signed release stating that it is okay to use their name)—or the ones you wanted to dump off the table—can be turned into stories for trade journals or for the dozens of New Age magazines that solicit those; many of them are regional, and they solicit personal growth experiences all the time. Even if you decide you can't personally write for anything except your journal right now, doing that will give you practice for writing other things—like advertisements and press releases that will help your business. Keeping a journal relating to your experiences as a massage therapist and a businessperson will serve you as a catalyst for new ideas, and a reminder not to repeat old mistakes. Taking those few minutes a day to do your writing will also serve as a stress-relieving activity for you. Make your goal to write in your journal, or set a goal to write for publication, and then follow through. And as someone who's already published, and who has received rejection letters, let me tell you that a rejection notice isn't the worst thing in the world. Most of the time, they'll give you a clue about why you were rejected—either the article just isn't something they're looking for at this particular time, or it's not up to their literary standards. The point is to *try*. All they can say is yes or no, and it might be yes!

Professional Presentation

If you have developed a new technique or a new twist on an old one, or conducted research as mentioned in Chapter 45, you can put that together into an interesting article. This is one instance where, in addition to using the spell-check, you may want to pay a professional editor to whip it into shape before you send it out to journals, unless you are very confident in your own abilities (if I didn't have a great editor, you wouldn't be reading this book!). As of press time, the going rate for professional editing is two to three dollars per page in most places, and it's definitely worth twenty dollars to get a ten-page article edited into professional sounding, easy to read condition. Of course, editors still have the right to edit, and they will, but they don't expect to have to copyedit articles for typos and incorrect grammar. They expect manuscripts to be professionally presented, and to follow whatever guidelines they have set up. If you are planning to submit to a journal or magazine, check on their website first; there is usually a page with submission guidelines. If you don't find them on the website, a phone call is in order before submitting anything. Some publications are very strict about what format the manuscript is in, what months they review submissions, what type of articles they are looking for, and so forth. Better to be prepared and not waste your time or theirs by submitting in the wrong way at the wrong time.

You may go that further step and decide to put your new technique, your research, or your personal experiences into a book. This chapter isn't meant to be a how-to on how to write a book, but a lesson for you: if you have always had that desire, why don't you act on it? Although I have previously had a book about massage published, the first novel that I wrote remains in a drawer unpublished—but I can't tell you how satisfied I was when I typed the last word of it, and I had then and still have years later the attitude that so what if it never gets published, I still have a book that I wrote.

Margaret's Story

I've always enjoyed writing. I decided to see if I could actually get something published, so I started with a little holistic healing magazine that is distributed locally. I was thrilled when they accepted my story about deciding to go to massage school at the ripe old age of 57. Since then, I've had two articles about massage published in regional health magazines. It's very exciting to see my name in print and my clients are impressed, too!

Mark Twain once said, "The secret of any overwhelming task is to break it down into a number of small tasks, and then start on the first one." If you don't write that first word, you'll never write the last one.

My Personal Journey

This Week's Activity: Getting Published Date____________________

For this week's activity, you are going to set the intention to get an article (or a book—doesn't hurt to think big!) published. Gather your journals and peruse them for ideas; look over your findings, if you've been doing research. Pretend you're back in school and your homework is to write a paper on any facet of massage and bodywork, whether that be technique, ethics, marketing, or whatever you feel you have a particular interest or amount of expertise in. It doesn't matter whether it's a trade journal, or just an interesting article about the benefits of massage for your local newspaper, *write something*. Then submit it! If it doesn't get accepted, you can always use it for your own newsletter.

My Goals

____

____

____

What's in my way?

____

____

____

What action can I take to remedy the situation?

____

____

____

One-Year Progress Update Date ____________________

____

____

____

POSITIVE AFFIRMATION: **My writing skills are becoming better all the time.**

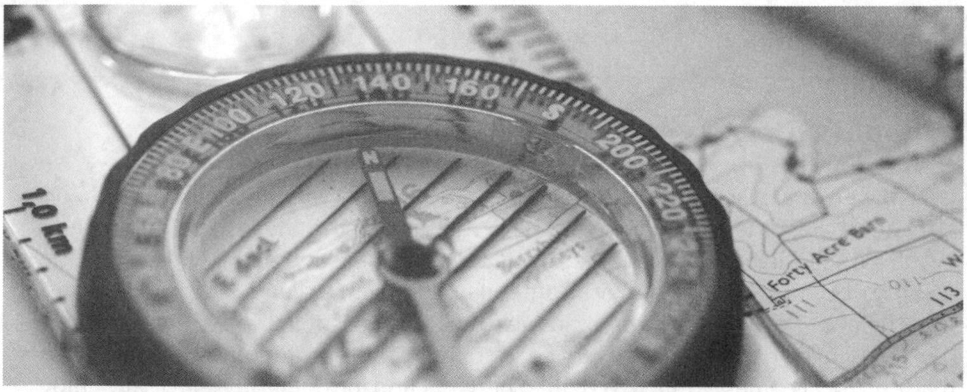

CHAPTER 48

Marketing to Athletes

Always bear in mind that your own resolution to succeed is more important than any one thing.

—Abraham Lincoln

There is a ready-made group of new clients right outside your door. They're everywhere in your town: at the gym, on the track, in the pool, in the wrestling ring, on the field, the golf course, and at the rodeo. They're athletes. Athletes injure themselves a lot, and they need rehabilitation. Even if they're not injured, they need a warm-up massage before competition, and a cool-down massage will help them avoid cramps. Massage can and should be part of their training program. It's up to you to make them wise to that fact. The best way to do that is by going where they are.

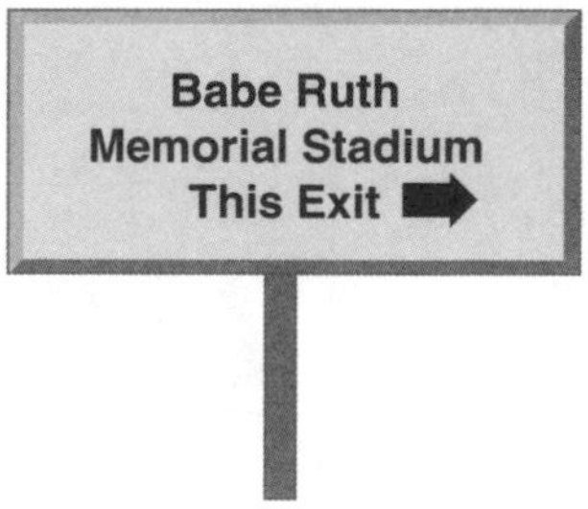

Approach a team manager, a coach, a gym owner, or other IPIC (Important Person in Charge) and tell them what you do. Go armed with your brochures on sports massage (these can be bought pre-printed or you can make your own) and business cards and ask permission to set up shop. A table will work better for sports massage than a chair. The athletes can remain clothed so there will be no need for linens; just bring a box of disinfectant wipes to clean the table between each person and a box of disposable face cradle covers.

Sports massage in the field is not about privacy or ambience. It's short sessions, 10 or 15 minutes at a dollar a minute, or whatever the going rate is in your area. You can set up in a shady spot near the field, under a tent, or in the corner of the gym if they don't have an empty room for you to work in. A percentage of what you make may go to the gym or the team. Settle those details with the contact person before you get started. If you live in a city that has a professional team, maybe you'll even apply for a job. You might become an official team massage therapist at a great salary, travel across the country, and receive big tips from the rich and famous. You'll never know if you don't apply.

My Story

Jimmy's Story

I'm a weekend warrior myself—love to play basketball with my buddies, try to do racquetball at the gym whenever I have the time, get in the occasional game of golf. When I first told my buddies I was going to massage school, they gave me some ribbing about it, but they all agreed to be practice clients. I've been licensed a little over a year and I almost exclusively do sports massage. I've got my brochures in every gym, given them to every coach of every team around, make it a point to attend local games as much as I can to network and introduce myself. I really enjoy my work. I feel like my clients see tangible results in their performance and feel good that I had a hand (no pun intended) in that.

Every Age and Stage

Doing sports massage at an event is a bonanza because you give a business card to every athlete, and while you're giving them their short massage, give them your prepared speech about regular massage being a part of their training program and enhancing their flexibility, stamina, and performance. Don't limit yourself. In addition to the serious athletes and the weekend warriors on the field, children participate in sports, and though they tend to bounce back a lot faster than adults, they do suffer injuries that would be helped by massage. People from eight to eighty-eight (and beyond) are golfers. A former colleague of mine used to market herself exclusively at golf courses by advertising that putting the body back in balance could lower your golf score. She was a very busy lady.

When you're out in the field, or at the track or the gym, take your appointment book with you so you can book appointments on the spot. It's a prime situation for booking people on a regular schedule. If they say they want to come Thursday at 4 pm, just ask if they would like to reserve that spot on a weekly or bi-weekly basis as a part of their regular training regimen. You may want to offer them a discount for booking *X* number of sessions in advance as an enticement.

My Personal Journey

This Week's Activity: Marketing to Athletes Date__________________

For this week's activity, you are going to market your services to athletes. If you're still a student, you might get your foot in the door by doing some community service on a sports team. If you're in practice, get out and introduce yourself to the sports community—visit the football field, the golf course, the tennis court, the track—wherever you can go in your area that are potential venues for sports massage. Take brochures and cards. Make some special flyers about sports massage and put them in as many athletic settings as you can.

My Goals

____

____

____

What's in my way?

____

____

____

What action can I take to remedy the situation?

____

____

____

One-Year Progress Update

____

____

____

POSITIVE AFFIRMATION: **Massaging athletes improves their performance and my prosperity.**

CHAPTER 49

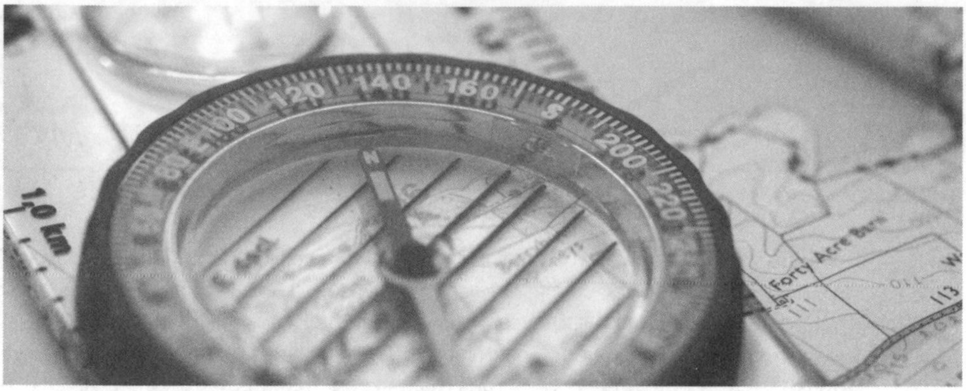

Start Your Own Support Group for Massage Therapists

The best way to succeed in life is to act on the advice that we give others.

—AUTHOR UNKNOWN

The big organizations such as AMTA and ABMP are great therapist support—and big! The meetings, while regular, are only a couple of times a year. A smaller, more intimate group of therapists getting together to eat, meet, swap massage, share ethical dilemmas, marketing ideas, meet new people to trade referrals with, and so forth sounds wonderful, doesn't it? If you don't know of a group like that in your area, don't sit around waiting for one to manifest. *You* be the one to start it.

My Story

Gerry's Story

I can't take the credit for starting my support group; someone invited me to join one and it's a great little group. I work in a resort spa where the pace is very fast and sometimes stressful, and it's good to have peer support. Others in the group are a good mix—several self-employed people, one who works in a chiropractor's office, one who works at a hospice. No one has an office big enough to accommodate everybody so we handle it a little differently. We all meet for supper in a nice restaurant once a month and everyone brings their appointment book, and we set up trades with each other. I think everybody gets a lot out of it. I know I do.

Collaboration, Not Competition

There are enough stressed-out people and aching bodies to go around. Fostering a spirit of collaboration, rather than competition, among other massage therapists is the way to success. Professional jealousy is not an attractive quality in any person. Rise above it.

A couple of years ago another therapist called and asked me to join a group she was starting. I thought it was a great idea! We get together about once every month or six weeks, taking turns meeting at each other's offices. Sometimes there are four, sometimes six or eight. We bring a covered dish or order pizza, or sometimes the hosting therapist provides the food and we all chip in a few dollars. After eating and meeting, we trade massage with each other. We are nurturing and supporting each other, we who are typically the caretakers.

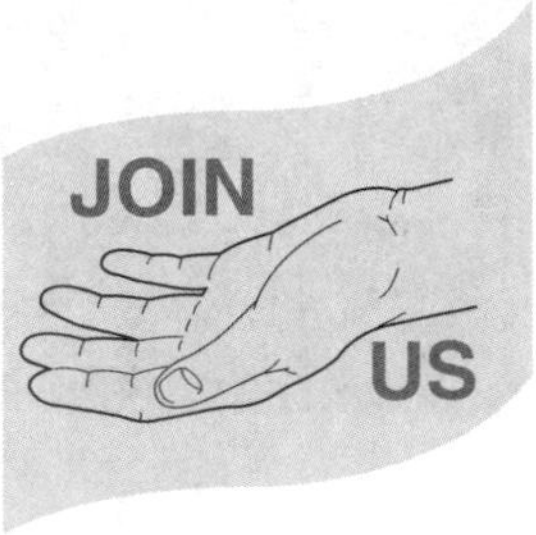

If you want to start a group, just look in the phone book and call the other therapists in town, or get their mailing address and send them an invitation. No expense to anyone other than the meal; a chance to network with people who understand your unique job challenges, and a free massage. You can't beat it. You might get a standoffish, competitive-type therapist or two who decline to join. Don't take it personally. It's not about you.

My Personal Journey

This Week's Activity: Starting a Massage Support Group

Date________________

For this week's activity, you are going to start a massage therapist's support group. If you're still a student, this might be a study group, too—get together, eat, study, and swap a massage with your classmates. If you're in practice, call or send an invitation to the other therapists in town. Host the first one at your office or even your home, if you don't have enough space for more than one massage table at your office. Make it at least a bi-monthly event.

My Goals

What's in my way?

What action can I take to remedy the situation?

One-Year Progress Update

Date________________

POSITIVE AFFIRMATION: **I support my colleagues and they support me.**

CHAPTER

50

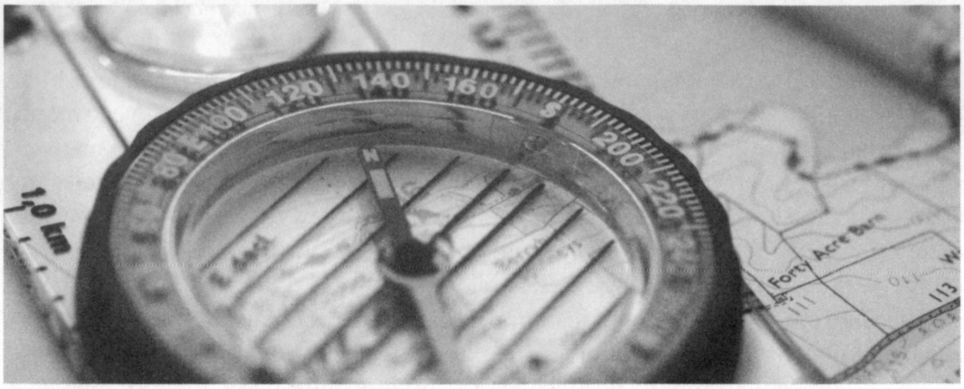

Be On Call

Some succeed because they are destined to, but most succeed because they are determined to.

—Henry Van Dyke

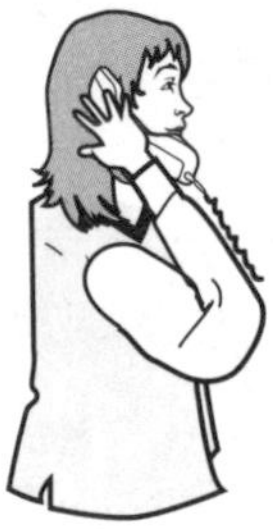

If you don't have your own business yet, or even if you do, but don't have as many customers as you want yet, consider being on call for other places. An enterprising therapist I know has visited every massage therapy business and spa within her county and the adjoining counties, and offered herself as an on-call therapist. She's made it plain to every business owner that she isn't looking for full-time work; she's ethical and doesn't try to take clients with her from one place to another or solicit them for herself; and she's available on a first-come, first-served basis. She's bailed me out a few times when a staff member was sick or on vacation, and she does the same for others.

How it Works

This enterprising woman might be at a chiropractor's office on Monday, a spa on Tuesday, my office on Wednesday, and somebody else's office the rest of the week. She's quite happy working this way, says it's never boring, and though she doesn't have a set schedule, she always manifests enough work to make a good living and keep herself happy with her myriad jobs. She turns down work and takes days off whenever the notion strikes. She works at a ritzy spa in Cape Cod during the summer months, and does her here-there-and-everywhere in North Carolina the rest of the year. Her massage table and supplies are always in her car; most places provide that for her, but she's prepared, just in case. She dresses professionally, is very personable, gives a great massage, and people are glad to get her services. This works very well for her. The first year or two she was licensed as a therapist, she found it hard for her to build a regular clientele in North Carolina since she only lives here half the year, so floating around to different businesses has been a smart choice for her.

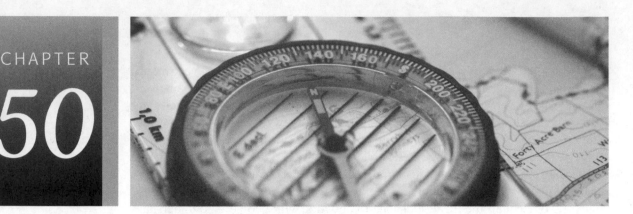

Ramona's Story

I've worked as an on-call therapist since I graduated from massage school about six years ago. I mainly rotate between several salons; they are smaller places where the owner does want to offer massage but doesn't really have enough demand to keep a therapist busy full-time. I have also covered for therapists who were sick, had a family emergency, or were just on vacation. I'm never bored, don't have any overhead, and can take time off work any time I want to, and I don't lose any business when I take off for Cape Cod in the summertime.

If you do have enough business at this point in time and don't have an interest in being on call yourself, but aren't yet in the position to take on a partner or hire someone to help you, you might consider using an on-call therapist to help with overflow. A student fresh out of school might be glad for the opportunity. You'll be helping someone and getting something you need in return.

My Personal Journey

This Week's Activity: Being on Call Date____________________

For this week's activity, you are going to either make an effort to do some work as an on-call therapist, or focus on finding a therapist who could be on call for you (or both). If you're about to graduate from massage school or just starting out, visit all the massage therapists around and offer your services as an on-call therapist. Let the owner know what skills you have, what equipment you are willing to transport, what days and hours you are on call, and so forth. Make sure they know you are ethical, interested in on-call work, and not trying to steal clients away to another business. Make up flyers advertising your on-call services to leave at the businesses you approach. If you could use the services of an on-call therapist but don't have one, try placing a cheap classified ad, or call the nearest massage school. Most schools maintain a list of available jobs for interested graduates.

My Goals

____

____

____

What's in my way?

____

____

____

What action can I take to remedy the situation?

____

____

____

One-Year Progress Update Date ____________________

____

____

____

POSITIVE AFFIRMATION: **I cultivate mutually advantageous relationships with other therapists.**

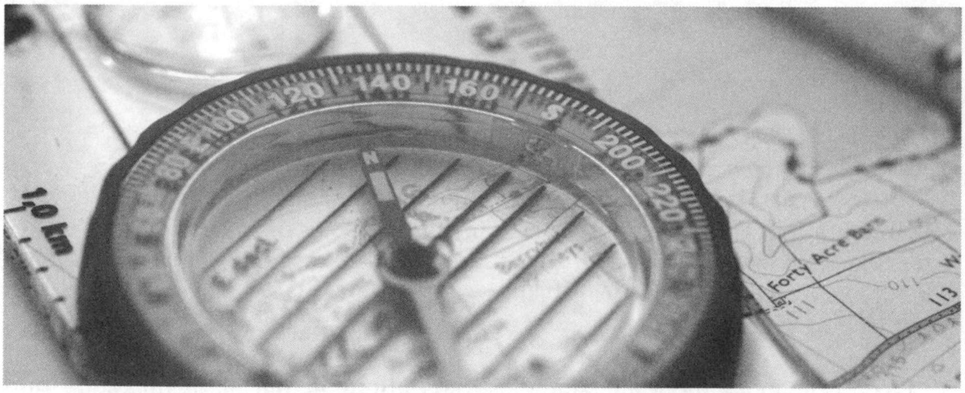

CHAPTER

51

Continuing Your Marketing Education

The guy who takes a chance, who walks the line between the known and the unknown, who is unafraid of failure, will succeed.

—Gordon Parks

One of the great benefits to learning as much as you can on the subject will be absorbing the knowledge and experience of people who have various circumstances—coming from different geographical areas, different populations, different work environments, different education, and so forth. Studying the perspective of others will give you new insight and new inspiration. Never stop learning! New ideas are born every day. Every day is a new opportunity for mental *and* financial growth.

Where to Learn

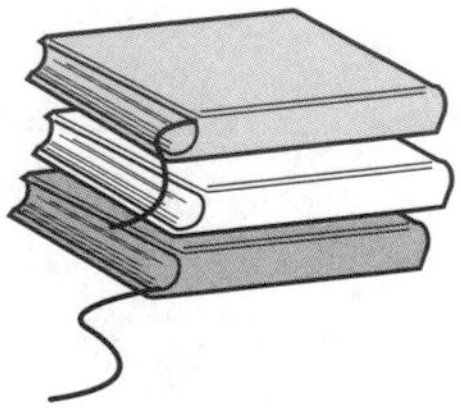

Yes, please go out and buy other authors' books. The marketing tactics that I have gone over in this book are the things that have worked for me. Other people are going to have different ideas that have worked for them. There will be disagreement between what they say and what I say. For instance, one book I read states "Giving away free massage will only get you customers that want free massage." I say that is hogwash, and my business records prove it—for me. Maybe that was *their* experience. In my belief system, what you give with a free heart will come back to you many, many times, and that has been *my* experience.

Attend as many marketing classes as you can; maybe even take a class in marketing at your local community college that isn't specific to massage but is just about marketing in general. Many merchant associations and chambers of commerce offer free or low-cost classes about marketing for the small business person. Take advantage of them. There are on-line courses and home-study classes you can take for continuing education credits. The Internet abounds with marketing websites; many of those are listed in Appendix IV.

My Story

Jack's Story

In the past year I have really gotten into attending marketing classes and reading marketing books, and the difference in my business has been amazing. Besides getting good marketing ideas, the most valuable part has been building my self confidence and faith in my own abilities.

One of the most important strategies for continuing your marketing education is to pick other businesses that are successful and that you admire and see what they're doing. The key is service. What makes the Ritz the Ritz or the Golden Door the gold standard? It's not just the opulent surroundings, although those are certainly nice—but it's the level of service. You don't have to be the Ritz in order to give top-drawer service. Let your focus be on continuing your education, continuing to grow as a massage therapist, and continuing to strive daily to improve your business and your level of service. If you abide by that philosophy, your business will practically market itself.

My Personal Journey

This Week's Activity: Continuing Your Marketing Education Date________________

For this week's activity, you are going to continue your marketing education. Peruse the Internet sites listed in Appendix IV. Go to the library and check out a marketing book; make a resolution to read one marketing book a month for the next year. Make it a point that one of the continuing education classes you attend this year will be about marketing. Visit a few successful businesses you admire and note what it is that makes them stand out to you, and what things they are doing marketing-wise.

My Goals

What's in my way?

What action can I take to remedy the situation?

One-Year Progress Update Date________________

POSITIVE AFFIRMATION: **Continuing my education is of great benefit to me.**

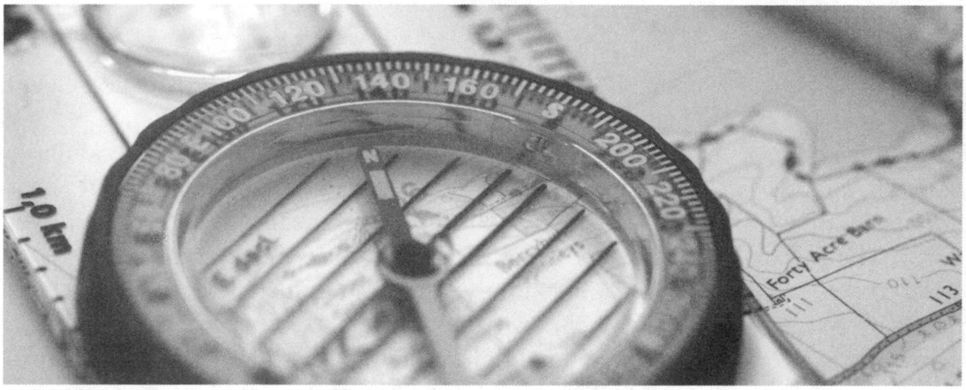

CHAPTER 52

Taking Stock: The Year in Review

People rarely succeed unless they have fun in what they are doing.
—Dale Carnegie

If you have followed the basic outline of this book, and done all or as many of the marketing activities that could fit your particular case, it's time to stop and take stock. As stated in the beginning, not all of these suggestions will fit everyone, but most will fit anyone. Hopefully, by keeping the journal at the end of each activity, you have found many ideas that will work for you, or have recognized what won't.

Don't Get in Your Way

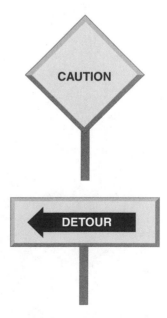

Procrastination is the biggest detriment to success. "I'll wait until next week to get my press release together." And somehow, next week never comes. Complacency is another: "I don't have to do anything; the clients I am meant to have will just wander in the door." Shyness, fear, lack of confidence in our own abilities, plain old laziness—so many things can interfere with prosperity; remember this: *whatever you allow to get in your way, will get in your way*. The main thing that gets in our way is ourselves.

You can make this book a five-year plan instead of a one-year plan if you want to—if you want to wait five years for success. The choice is yours. If you go to work every day with the intent of doing *something* to market your business, and you follow through with the *action* necessary to make that intent a reality, it will come a lot quicker.

Action is the key word. The newspapers and the radio stations are not going to call you to ask you if you have a press release or if anything new and exciting is happening at your business. Clients are not going to line up at the door for your special package if they don't know you have it. The *action* has to come from you. If the year has passed, and you are no better off than you were when it began, be brutally honest with yourself about why that is. Don't blame luck. Don't blame Providence. Don't play shame and blame at all—but look within.

Things do happen that are beyond our control; family tragedies such as illness or death, our own health problems, or a child with special needs demands our attention. Sometimes you have to pick yourself up, dust yourself off, and start all over again. The rewards of this business are often more than monetary. Nothing is as satisfying as seeing someone hobble into your office, grimacing and stooped with pain, and an hour later, seeing them walk out with a relaxed posture and a smile on their face. Ask them for a testimonial before they get out the door! There are so many opportunities for success every day; the secret is to recognize them, grab them, and not let them pass you by.

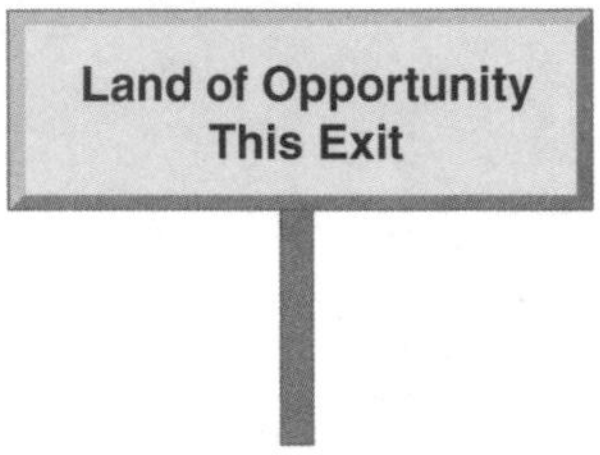

Succeeding in business is so much more than showing up for work every day. It's also recognizing your shortcomings, and taking whatever *action* you can to fix them. It's making adjustments where needed. It's asking for help and advice when you feel stuck or overwhelmed. It's taking care of your business and taking care of yourself. It's giving back to your community, and being a vital part of your community. It's having people think well of you. It's showing gratitude for what you have, and gracious acceptance of gratitude when it comes your way. It's being fair-minded, and not taking it personally any time something doesn't go your way. It's being prepared. It's believing in yourself and believing that you deserve to be successful. Remember, if you expect to fail, you've taken the first step on the path to failure. If you expect to succeed—and you take *action*—you've taken the first step on the path to success. Believe it!

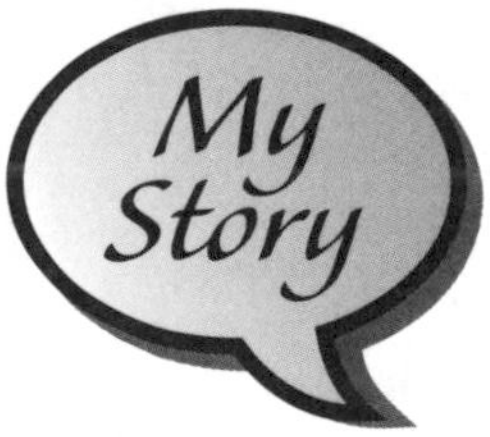

Laura's Story

More than a year has passed since I proposed this book to the publisher. By the time this is printed, I will have passed the fourth anniversary in my business, and it has been a joy and a challenge to go from where I started to where I am now. In looking back over my own journal, I have performed forty-six of the activities that I recommend in this book over the past twelve months. I didn't get around to having the guy in the Big Bird suit in front of the business this year and I wimped out on Halloween, but I'm making it a priority for next year! We are still exceeding my goal of getting one new customer a day every day of the year, and I am still doing *something* to market my business every day of the year, as much and as cheaply as possible. Business has increased—while advertising costs have decreased—as the amount of word of mouth marketing has continued to increase. Yours will do the same thing if you *practice taking action*. Happy marketing!

My Personal Journey

This Week's Activity: The Year in Review Date__________________

For this week's activity, you are going to take stock of the things you have done in the past year to increase your business. Go back through the book and count; there were 51 weeks of activities for you to do; how many did you actually do? How much effort did you put forth? If you were already in business and had the previous years' financial reports to compare to, you should do that, so you can see the improvement in black and white. Formulate your plan for next year; any of these ideas that you didn't do this year, resolve to do them in the next twelve months, and track your results.

My Goals

What's in my way?

What action can I take to remedy the situation?

One-Year Progress Update Date __________________

POSITIVE AFFIRMATION: **I embrace the responsibility for my own success.**

PART 4

Trip Tips: Resources for Massage Therapists

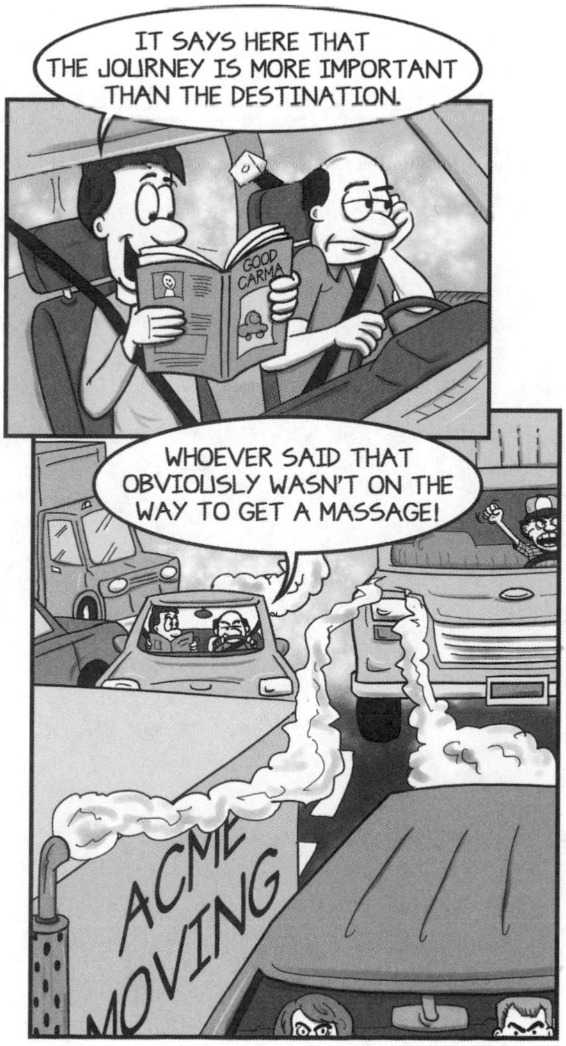
IT SAYS HERE THAT THE JOURNEY IS MORE IMPORTANT THAN THE DESTINATION.
GOOD CARMA
WHOEVER SAID THAT OBVIOUSLY WASN'T ON THE WAY TO GET A MASSAGE!
ACME MOVING

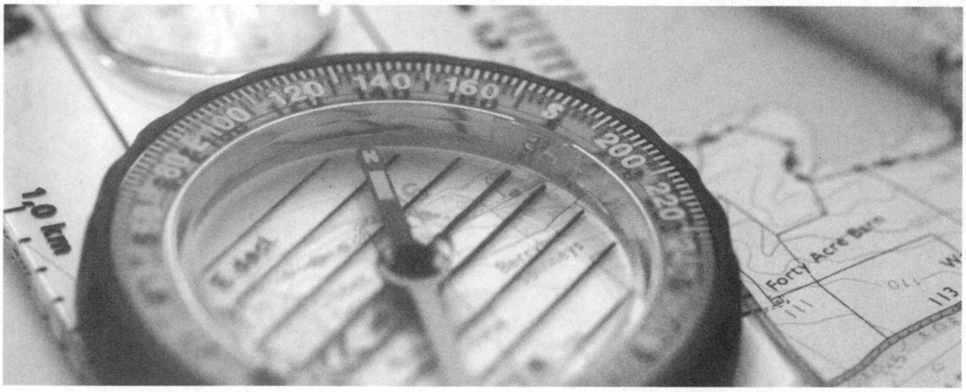

Introduction to the Appendices

Appendix I is a listing of state massage therapy boards and the contact information for those states that are regulating massage. Call, write, or visit the website for information pertaining to the requirements for licensure and other rules and regulations. You'll note that many of them do not have an e-mail address listed; that is because the address provided was for a specific individual. Please visit the website for the most current person to address e-mail to, should you decide to contact them that way.

Appendix II is a listing of the national professional associations for massage therapy and bodywork. Appendix III contains sources for marketing materials for the massage therapy profession; Appendix IV is a listing of Internet resources for marketing massage, and Appendix V is a marketing calendar—a list of real and silly holidays, important days in history, and so forth that you can utilize to help plan promotions. Appendix VI is a list of other marketing books you might want to read.

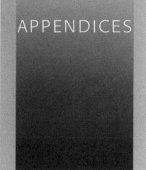

APPENDIX I

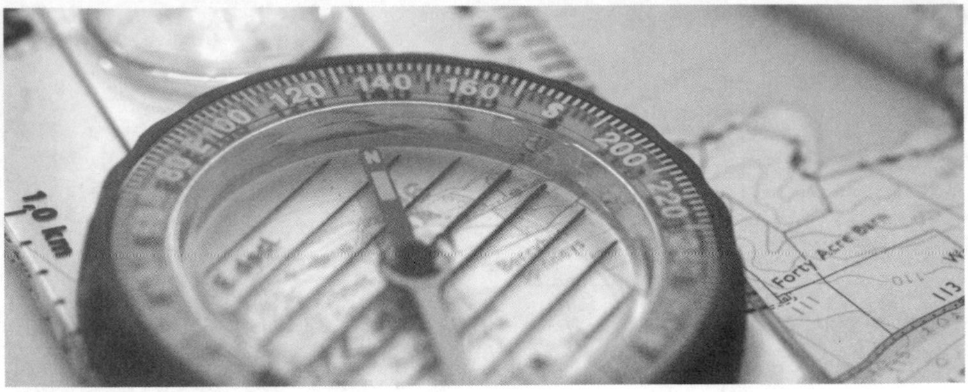

State Massage Therapy Boards

State of Alabama
Board of Massage Therapy
610 S. McDonough Street
Montgomery, AL 36104
334-269-9990 or
866-873-4664
334-263-6115 (fax)
Website: http://www.almtbd.state.al.us
E-mail: ALMTBD@aol.com

State of Arizona
Board of Massage Therapy
1400 West Washington, Suite #230
Phoenix, AZ 85007
602-542-8604
602-542-3093 (fax)
Website: http://www.massagetherapy.az.gov
E-mail: info@massageboard.state.az.us

State of Arkansas
Board of Massage Therapy
Post Office Box 20739
Hot Springs, AR 71903
501-520-0555
501-623-4130 (fax)
Website: http://www.arkansasmassagetherapy.com
E-mail: info@arkansasmassagetherapy.com

State of California
As of press time has no state licensure board for massage therapy.

State of Colorado
As of press time has no state licensure board for massage therapy.

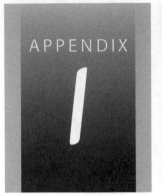

State of Connecticut
Connecticut Department of Public Health
Massage Therapist Licensure
410 Capitol Ave.
Post Office Box 340308
Hanford, CT 06134
Website: http://www.dph.state.ct.us/Licensure/apps/PLIS/MassageTherapist
E-mail: oplc.dph@po.state.ct.us

State of Delaware
Board of Massage & Bodywork
Cannon Building, Suite 203
861 Silver Lake Blvd.
Dover, DE 19904
800-464-4357
302-739-2711 (fax)
Website: http://dpr.delaware.gov/boards/massagebodyworks/index.shtml
E-mail: see website for current e-mail.

State of Florida
Board of Massage Therapy
Post Office Box 6330
Tallahassee, FL 32314
850-245-4161
Website: http://www.doh.state.fl.us/mqa/massage/index.html
E-mail: MedicalQualityAssurance@doh.state.fl.us

State of Georgia
Board of Massage Therapy
237 Coliseum Drive
Macon, GA 31217
478-207-2440
478-207-1354 (fax)
Website: www.sos.state.ga.us/plb/massage
E-mail: see website for current e-mail.

State of Hawaii
DCCA-PVL
Attn: Massage
Post Office Box 3469
Honolulu, HA 96801
808-586-2694
Website: http://www.hawaii.gov/dcca/areas/pvl/boards/massage
E-mail: massage@dcca.hawaii.gov

State of Idaho
As of press time has no state licensure board for massage therapy.

State of Illinois
Massage Licensing Board
320 West Washington St.
Springfield, IL 62786

217-785-0800
Website: http://www.idfpr.com/dpr/who/masst.asp
E-mail: see website for current e-mail.

State of Indiana
As of press time has no state licensure board for massage therapy.

State of Iowa
Iowa Board of Massage Therapy Examiners
Lucas State Office Bldg.
321 E. 12th Street
Des Moines, IA 50319
585-281-6959
E-mail: see website for current e-mail.

State of Kansas
As of press time has no state licensure board for massage therapy.

State of Kentucky
Board of Massage Therapy
Post Office Box 1360
Frankfort, KY 40602
502-564-3296 ext. 240
502-564-4818 (fax)
Website: http://finance.ky.gov/ourcabinet/caboff/OAS/op/massth/
E-mail: see website for current e-mail.

State of Louisiana
Board of Massage Therapy
12022 Plank Rd.
Baton Rouge, LA 70811
225-771-4090
225-771-4021 (fax)
Website: http://www.lsbmt.org/
E-mail: admin@lsbmt.org

State of Maine
Office of Licensing and Registration
Massage Therapy
35 State House Station
Augusta, ME 04333
207-624-8613
207-624-8637 (fax)
Website: http://www.maine.gov/pfr/professionallicensing/professions/massage/
E-mail: see website for current e-mail.

State of Maryland
Maryland Board of Chiropractic Examiners
Massage Therapy Advisory Committee
4201 Patterson Avenue
Baltimore, MD 21215
410-764-4738

Website: http://www.mdmassage.org/
E-mail: see website for current e-mail.

State of Massachusetts
Board of Registration of Massage Therapy
617-727-3074
Website: www.mass.gove/dpl/boards/mt/index.htm
*As of press time, this Board is in the process of forming and is seeking members, and as of yet has no permanent address. Massage therapists should apply for licensure in their own community, according to the website.
E-mail: see website for current e-mail.

State of Michigan
As of press time has no state licensure board for massage therapy.

State of Minnesota
As of press time has no state licensure board for massage therapy.

State of Mississippi
Board of Massage Therapy
Post Office Box 12489
Jackson, MS 39236
601-919-1517
601-919-1432 (fax)
Website: http://www.msbmt.state.ms.us/msbmt/msbmt.nsf
E-mail: director@msbmt.state.ms.us

State of Missouri
Board of Therapeutic Massage
3605 Missouri Blvd.
Post Office Box 1335
Jefferson City, MO 65102
573-522-6277
573-751-0735 (fax)
Website: http://pr.mo.gov/massage.asp
E-mail: massagether@pr.mo.gov

State of Montana
As of press time has no state licensure board for massage therapy.

State of Nebraska
Department of Health and Human Services—Regulation and Licensure
Credentialing Division
Post Office Box 94986
Lincoln, NE
402-471-2115
402-471-3577 (fax)
Website: http://www.hhs.state.ne.us/crl/mhcs/mass
E-mail: see website for current e-mail.

State of Nevada
Board of Massage Therapy
1755 E. Plumb Lane, Suite 252

Reno, NV 89502
775-668-1888
775-786-4264 (fax)
Website: http://www.massagetherapy.nv.gov/
E-mail: nvmassagebd@state.nv.us

State of New Hampshire
DHHS Office of Program Support
Licensing and Regulative Services
129 Pleasant St.
Concord, NH 03301
603-271-0277
603-271-5590 (fax)
Website: http://www.dhhs.nh.gov/DHHS/LRS/ELIGIBILITY/massage-license.htm
E-mail: see website for current e-mail.

State of New Jersey
New Jersey Board of Nursing
Attn: Massage, Bodywork, and Somatic Therapy
Post Office Box 45010
Newark, NJ 07101
973-504-6430
973-648-3481 (fax)
Website: http://www.state.nj.us/lps/ca/nursing/mass.htm
E-mail: see website for current e-mail.

State of New Mexico
Massage Therapy Board
2550 Cerrillos Rd.
Santa Fe, NM 87505
505-476-4870
Website: http://www.rld.state.nm.us/b&c/Massage/index.htm
E-mail: massage.board@state.nm.us

State of New York
Office of the Professions/Massage Therapy
State Education Building, 2nd Floor
Albany, NY 12234
518-474-3817, ext. 150
518-486-2981 (fax)
Website: http://www.op.nysed.gov/contact.htm
E-mail: msthbd@mail.nysed.gov

State of North Carolina
Board of Massage & Bodywork Therapy
Post Office Box 2539
Raleigh, NC 27602
919-546-0050
919-833-1059 (fax)
Website: www.bmbt.org
E-mail: admin@bmbt.org

State of North Dakota
Board of Massage
Post Office Box 218
Beach, ND 58621
701-872-4895
Website: http://www.ndboardofmassage.com/
E-mail: see website for current e-mail.

State of Ohio
State Medical Board of Ohio
Massage Therapy Advisory Committee
77 South High St., 17th Floor
Columbus, Ohio 43215
614-466-3934
614-728-5946 (fax)
Website: http://www.med.ohio.gov/mt_about_massage_therapy.htm
E-mail: see website for current e-mail.

State of Oklahoma
As of press time has no state licensure board for massage therapy.

State of Oregon
Board of Massage Therapists
748 Hawthorne Ave. NE
Salem, OR 97301
503-365-8657
503-385-4465 (fax)
Website: http://www.oregonmassage.org/
E-mail: see website for current e-mail.

State of Pennsylvania
As of press time has no state licensure board for massage therapy.

State of Rhode Island
Office of Health Professions Regulation
Massage Therapist Licensing
3 Capitol Hill, Room 105
Providence, RI 02908
401-222-2827
401-222-1272 (fax)
Website: http://www.health.ri.gov/hsr/professions/massage.php
E-mail: see website for current e-mail.

State of South Carolina
Board of Massage/Bodywork Therapy
Post Office Box 11329
Columbia, SC 29210
803-896-4490
803-896-4484 (fax)
Website: http://www.llr.state.sc.us/POL/MassageTherapy/
E-mail: see website for current e-mail.

State of Tennessee
Board of Massage Licensure
227 French Landing, Suite 300
Nashville, TN 37243
515-532-3202
Website: http://www2.state.tn.us/health/Boards/Massage/
E-mail: TN.health@state.tn.us

State of Texas
Department of State Health Services
Massage Therapy Licensing
100 West 49th St.
Austin, TX 78756
888-963-7111
Website: http://www.dshs.state.tx.us/massage/
E-mail: see website for current e-mail.

State of Utah
Board of Massage
160 East 300 South, 1st Floor Lobby
Salt Lake City, UT 84111
801-520-6628
801-530-6511 (fax)
Website: http://www.dopl.utah.gov/licensing/massage.html
E-mail: see website for current e-mail.

State of Virginia
Board of Nursing
Attn: Massage Therapy Certification
6603 West Broad St., 5th Fl.
Richmond, VA 23230
804-662-9909
804-662-9512 (fax)
Website: www.dhp.virginia.gov
E-mail: see website for current e-mail.

State of Washington
Washington State Department of Health
Health Professions Quality Assurance
Post Office Box 47865
Olympia, WA 98504
360-236-4700
Website: www.doh.wa.gov/massage
E-mail: hpqa.csc@doh.wa.gov

Washington, D.C.
Department of Health
Board of Massage Therapy
717 14th St. NW
Washington, DC 2005
877-672-2174
202-727-8471 (fax)
Website: www.dchealth.dc.gov
E-mail: see website for current e-mail.

State of West Virginia
Massage Therapy Licensure Board
704 Bland Street
Box 107
Suite 308
Bluefield, WV 24701
304-325-5862
Website: www.wvmassage.org
E-mail: see website for current e-mail.

State of Wisconsin
Massage Therapists and Body Worker Council
Bureau of Health Service Professions
1400 E. Washington Ave.
Post Office Box 8935
Madison, WI 53708
608-266-2102
Website: http://drl.wi.gov/boards/mtb/index.htm
E-mail: web@drl.state.wi.us

State of Wyoming
As of press time has no state licensure board for massage therapy.

APPENDIX 11

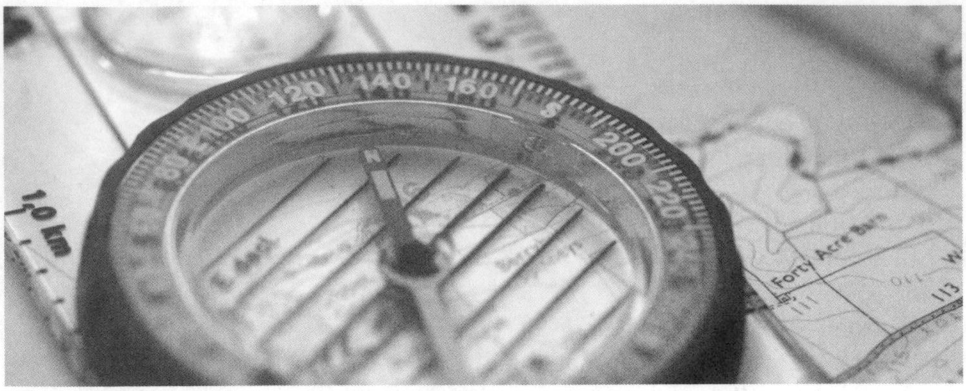

Massage and Bodywork Associations

The following are some of the associations for practitioners of massage and bodywork located in the United States. There are many international organizations as well. Many specific modalities also have their own associations; only the major ones are listed here.

American Massage Therapy Association
500 Davis Street, Suite 900
Evanston, IL 60201-4695
Toll-Free: 1-877-905-2700
Phone: 847-864-0123
Fax: 847-864-1178
E-mail: info@amtamassage.org
Website: http://www.amtamassage.org
Note that AMTA has chapters in every state. You can find your state chapter on the main website.

American Massage Council
1851 East First Street, Suite 1160
Santa Ana, CA 92705
Phone: 800-500-3930
Fax: 714-571-1863
E-mail: info@massagecouncil.com
Website: http://www.massagecouncil.com

American Medical Massage Association
1845 Lakeshore Drive, Suite 7
Muskegon, MI 49441
Phone: 888-375-7245
Fax: 231-755-2963
E-mail: info@americanmedicalmassage.com
Website: http://www.americanmedicalmassage.com

Ancient Healing Arts Association
POB 1785
Bensalem, PA 19020
Phone: 866-843-2422
Fax: 305-402-3134
E-mail: Healers@ancienthealingarts.org
Website: http://ancienthealingarts.org

Associated Bodywork and Massage Professionals
1271 Sugarbush Drive
Evergreen, CO 80439
Phone: 800-458-2267 * 303-674-8478
Fax: 800-667-8260
E-mail: expectmore@abmp.com
Website: http://www.abmp.com

CMTA, Clinical Massage Therapy Association, Inc.
3000 Connecticut Avenue, NW, Suite 102
Washington, D.C. 20008
Phone: 877-221-3444
Fax: 202-332-0531

FSMBT, Federation of State Massage Therapy Boards
7111 W 151st Street, Suite 356
Overland Park, KS 66223
Phone: 913-681-0380
Fax: 913-681-0391
Toll free: 888-70FSMTB
Email: info@fsmtb.org
Website: www.fsmtb.org

International Association of Healthcare Practitioners
11211 Prosperity Farms Road, Suite D-325
Palm Beach Gardens, FL 33410
Phone: 800-311-9204 561-622-4334
Fax: 561-622-4771
E-mail: iahp@iahp.com
Website: http://www.iahp.com

IMA Group, International Massage Association, Inc.
P.O. Drawer 421
Warrenton, VA 20188-0421
Phone: 540-351-0800
Fax: 540-351-0816
E-mail: info@imagroup.com
Website: www.imagroup.com

National Association of Nurse Massage Therapists
P.O. Box 24004
Huber Heights, OH 45424
Phone: 800-262-4017
E-mail: nanmtadmin@nanmt.org
Website: http://www.nanmt.org

National Certification Board for Therapeutic Massage and Bodywork
1901 S. Meyers Road, Suite 240
Oakbrook Terrace, IL 60181
Phone: 800-296-0664 630-627-8000
Fax: 866-402-1890
E-mail: info@ncbtmb.com
Website: http://www.ncbtmb.com

United States Medical Massage Association
POB 2394
Surf City, NC 28445
Phone: 888-322-5520
E-mail: info@usmedicalmassage.org
Website: http://www.usmedicalmassage.org

For Practitioners of Specific Modalities

American CranioSacral Therapy Association
The Upledger Institute
11211 Prosperity Farms Road, Suite D-325
Palm Beach Gardens, FL 33410
Phone: 561-622-4334
Fax: 561-622-4771
E-mail: upledger@upledger.com
Website: http://www.acsta.com

American Polarity Therapy Association
122 North Elm Street, Suite 512
Greensboro, NC 27401
Phone: 336-574-1121
Fax: 336-574-1151
E-mail: hq@polaritytherapy.org
Website: http://www.polaritytherapy.org

Guild for Structural Integration
3107 28th Street
Boulder, CO 80301
Phone: 303-447-0122
Fax: 303-447-4815
E-mail: info@rolfguild.org
Website: www.rolfguild.org

International Association of Infant Massage
1891 Goodyear Avenue, Suite 622
Ventura, CA 93003
Phone: 805-644-8524
E-mail: IAIM4US@aol.com
Website: http://www.iaim.ws/home.html

International Thai Therapists Association
POB 1048
Palm Springs, CA 92263
Phone: 760-641-0756
E-mail: itta@core.com
Website: http://www.thaimassage.com

Lymphology Association of North America
P.O. Box 466
Wilmette, IL 60091
Phone: 773-756-8971
E-mail: lana@clt-lana.org
Website: http://www.clt-lana.org

Reflexology Association of America
4012 Rainbow Ste. K-PMB#585
Las Vegas, NV 89103-2059
E-mail: http://www.reflexology-usa.org/contact_us.htm
Website: http://www.reflexology-usa.org

Rhythmical Massage Association of North America
15 Manhan St.
Northampton, MA 01060
E-mail: esustick@hotmail.com
Website: http://www.artemisia.net/rmta

US Sports Massage Federation
2156 Newport Boulevard
Costa Mesa, CA 92627
Phone: 949-642-0735

United States Trager Association
13801 W. Center St., Ste. C
POB 1009
Burton, OH 44021
Phone: 440-834-0308
Fax: 440-834-0365
E-mail: info@trager-us.org
Website: http://www.trager-us.org

The Zero Balancing Health Association
Kings Contrivance Village Center
8640 Guilford Road, Suite 240
Columbia MD 21046
Phone: 410-381-8956
Fax: 410-381-9634
E-mail: zbaoffice@zerobalancing.com
Website: http://www.zerobalancing.com

APPENDIX III

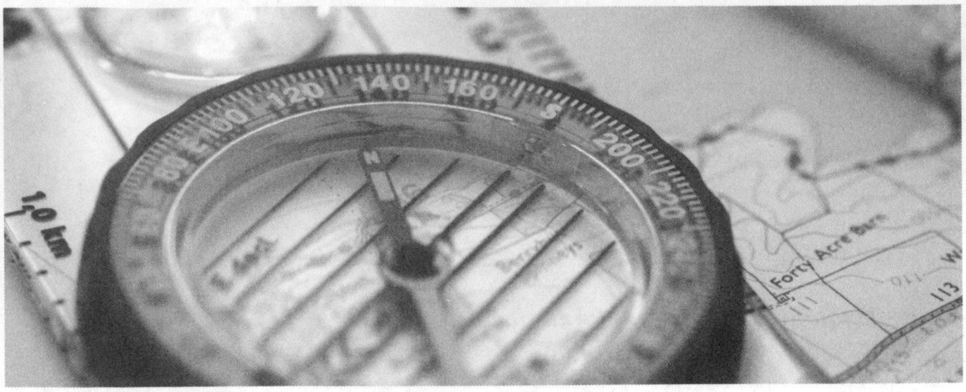

Marketing Materials for Massage Therapists

The following companies provide high-quality printed business forms, newsletters, marketing materials, and promotional items specific to the massage industry. There are many others, but these are companies I have personally dealt with in the past and know to be reliable and provide a good value for the money.

Here's The Rub
66 Evergreen Avenue
Warminster, PA 18974
Phone: 877-484-3782
E-mail: laura@herestherub.net
Website: http://www.herestherub.net

Information 4 People, Inc.
POB 1038
Olympia, WA 98507-1038
Phone: 800-754-9790
Fax: 360-705-3864
E-mail: info@info4people.com
Website: http://info4people.com

Staying in Touch Newsletters
Massage Marketing
221 North Third Street
Thayer, MO 65791
Phone: 877-634-1010
E-mail: jonlum@centurytel.net
Website: http://shoppingcarts4you.com/massagemarketing

Massage Warehouse
9005 N. Industrial Rd
Peoria, IL 61615-1511
Phone: 770-810-2680
Website: www.massagewarehouse.com

Vista Print
100 Hayden Avenue
Lexington, MA 02421
Phone: 800-961-2075
Website: http://www.vistaprint.com

Watercolors, Inc.
POB 6269
Navarre, FL 32566
Phone: 800-804-2019
Fax: 850-936-9561
E-mail: massage@watercolorscards.com
Website: http://www.watercolorscards.com

APPENDIX IV

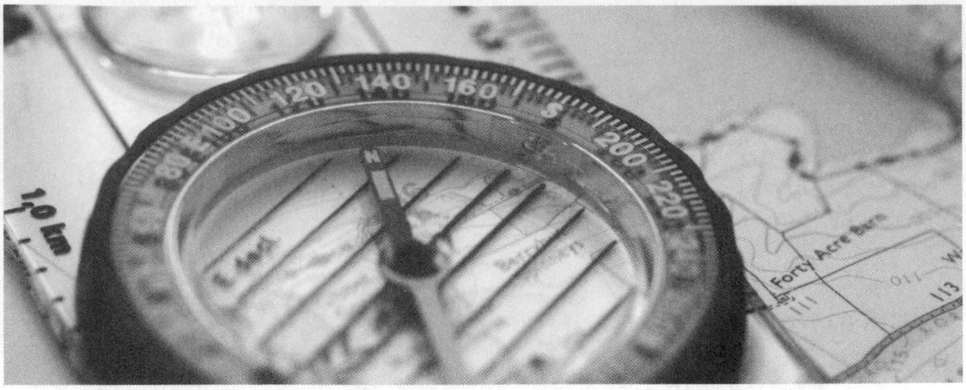

Internet Resources for Marketing Massage

There are dozens, if not hundreds, of places on the Internet where you can place a listing for free or for a minimal charge. There are also many places that will give you a reciprocal link—but be careful and do not link to any places that also link to adult websites, sexual content, etc. There are also a lot of websites with helpful marketing tips for therapists; many also include listing pages.

Here are some of the top ones:

http://www.massagedirect.com/marketing.htm
http://www.thebodyworker.com/marketingintro.html
http://www.bodyzone.com
http://www.newagemarketingtips.com
http://www.massagenetwork.com
http://www.amtamassage.org/findamassage/locator.htm
http://www.abmp.com
http://www.massageontheweb.com
http://www.massage-classifieds.com
http://www.massageoutpost.com

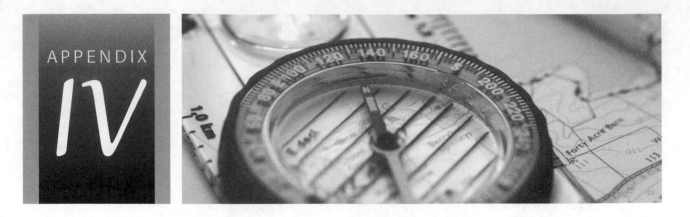

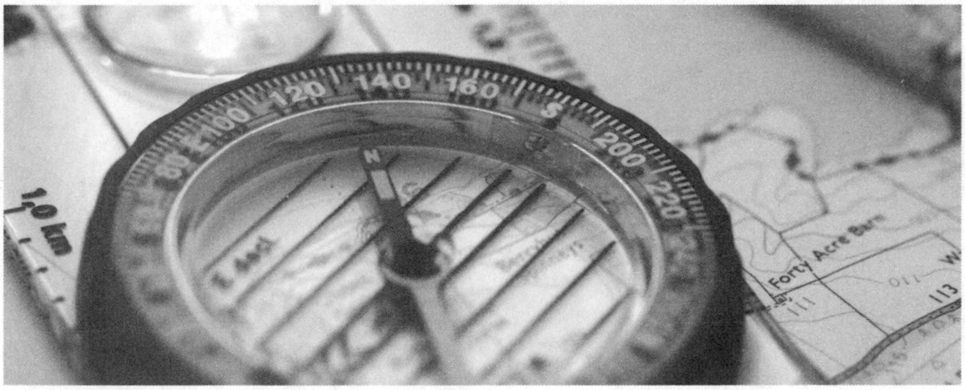

APPENDIX V

Marketing Calendar

January

January is International Business Success Resolutions Month.

1. New Year's Day
2. Science Fiction Day
3. National Write to Congress Day
4. Trivia Day
5. Second-Hand Wardrobe Day
6. Traditional Twelfth Night
7. Toss Out Your Fruitcake Day
8. Women's Day
9. National Clean Off Your Desk Day
10. Day in History: First meeting of the United Nations
11. Alexander Hamilton's Birthday
12. Recycle the Christmas Tree Day
13. International Skeptics Day
14. Penguin Awareness Day
15. World Religion Day
16. Martin Luther King's Birthday
17. Customer Service Day
18. Winnie the Pooh Day
19. Women's Healthy Weight Day
20. Inauguration Day
21. National Hugging Day
22. Celebrate Life Day
23. National Pie Day
24. National Speak Up and Succeed Day
25. National Pay a Compliment Day
26. National Peanut Brittle Day
27. Have Fun at Work Day
28. Day in History: The first ski lift in America opened in Vermont
29. Free Thinkers Day
30. Bubble Wrap Appreciation Day

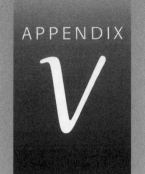

February

February is National Black History Month.

1. Women's Heart Health Day
2. Ground Hog Day
3. Wear Red Day
4. USO Day
5. Weather Person's Day
6. Bob Marley Day
7. Leadership Success Day
8. Boy Scout Day
9. Day in History: Volleyball was invented (1895)
10. World Marriage Day
11. National Shut-in Visitation Day
12. Men's Day
13. Day in History: First public school in America founded in Boston (1635)
14. Valentine's Day
15. Gummy Bear Day
16. Day in History: The first 9-1-1 emergency number in service (1968)
17. Random Acts of Kindness Day
18. Day in History: Elm Farm Ollie becomes first cow to fly in a plane (1930)
19. Chocolate Mint Day
20. North American Hoodie Hoo Day
21. Single Tasking Day
22. Inconvenience Yourself Day
23. National Chili Day
24. Day in History: National Public Radio is founded (1970)
25. Day in History: 16th Amendment ratified allowing income tax (1913)
26. For Pete's Sake Day
27. International Polar Bear Day
28. Tooth Fairy Day

March

March is American Red Cross Month.

1. Stop Bad Service Day
2. World Book Day
3. World Day of Prayer
4. Scrapbooking Day
5. Healing From the Inside Out Day
6. Day in History: Bayer registered *aspirin* as a trademark
7. Day in History: Alexander Graham Bell patented the telephone (1876)
8. International Working Women's Day
9. Panic Day
10. Middle Name Pride Day
11. Genealogy Day
12. Girl Scout Day
13. Good Samaritan Day
14. Pi Day
15. The Ides of March

16. Day in History: First liquid-fuel rocket launch (1926)
17. Companies That Care Day
18. Awkward Moments Day
19. Day in History: Daylight Savings Time is approved by Congress (1918)
20. National Agriculture Day
21. Memory Day
22. National Common Courtesy Day
23. Near Miss Day
24. National Chocolate Covered Raisins Day
25. Pecan Day
26. Legal Assistant's Day
27. Kite Flying Day
28. American Diabetes Association Alert Day
29. National Mom & Pop Business Owner's Day
30. Doctor's Day
31. Bunsen Burner Day

April

April is International Customer Loyalty Month.

1. April Fool's Day
2. Check Your Batteries Day
3. National Workplace Napping Day
4. World Rat Day
5. School Librarian Apprcciation Day
6. National Have Fun at Work Day
7. World Health Day
8. Tutor Appreciation Day
9. Winston Churchill Day
10. National Sibling Day
11. Babershop Quartet Day
12. National Licorice Day
13. International Plant Appreciation Day
14. Pan American Day
15. Husband Appreciation Day
16. Day in History: Apollo 16 leaves earth bound for the moon (1972)
17. Day in History: The Ford Motor Company debuts the Mustang (1964)
18. National Stress Awareness Day
19. Bicycle Day
20. Day in History: Sound is added to film for the first time (1926)
21. Day in History: Henry VIII becomes King of England (1509)
22. Earth Day
23. World Book & Copyright Day
24. Day in History: The Hubble space telescope is launched (1990)
25. Red Hat Society Day
26. Secretary's Day
27. Take Your Children to Work Day
28. Arbor Day
29. World T'ai Chi and QiGong Day
30. National Honesty Day

May

May is Fibromyalgia Education and Awareness Month.

1. May Day
2. Fire Day
3. Lumpy Rug Day
4. Respect for Chickens Day
5. Cinco de Mayo
6. Pun Day
7. Embrace Diversity Day
8. World Red Cross Day
9. National Teacher's Day
10. Donate a Day's Wages to Charity Day
11. Eat What You Want Day
12. Receptionists Day
13. National Babysitter's Day
14. National Dance Like a Chicken Day
15. National Chocolate Chip Day
16. National Sea Monkey Day
17. Pack Rat Day
18. Visit Your Relatives Day
19. Hug Your Cat Day
20. Armed Forces Day
21. National Waitstaff Day
22. Day in History: The toothpaste tube was invented (1892)
23. Penny Day
24. Brother's Day
25. National Tap Dancing Day
26. Grey Day
27. International Jazz Day
28. National Hamburger Day
29. Day in History: John F. Kennedy is born (1917)
30. Day in History: First observance of Memorial Day (1868)
31. National Seniors Health and Fitness Day

June

June is Entrepreneur's Do-It-Yourself Marketing Month.

1. Artists of America Day
2. Leave Work Early Day
3. Doughnut Day
4. National Cancer Survivors Day
5. World Environment Day
6. National Hunger Awareness Day
7. National Chocolate Ice Cream Day
8. Day in History: The first car is stolen in America (1896)
9. Donald Duck Day
10. National Yo-Yo Day
11. National Hug Day
12. Machine Day
13. National Juggling Day

14. Flag Day
15. Nursing Assistants Day
16. Fudge Day
17. Vinegar Day
18. National Splurge Day
19. Garfield the Cat Day
20. Ice Cream Soda Day
21. World Vegan Day
22. National Chocolate Éclair Day
23. National Take Your Dog to Work Day
24. Day in History: Henry VIII becomes King of England (1509)
25. Log Cabin Day
26. International Day Against Drug Abuse
27. National Columnists Day
28. Paul Bunyan Day
29. National Hand Shake Day
30. Day in History: *Gone With the Wind* published (1936)

July

July is National Hot Dog Month.

1. Build a Scarecrow Day
2. I Forgot Day
3. Air Conditioning Appreciation Day
4. Independence Day
5. Workaholics Day
6. National Fried Chicken Day
7. Chocolate Day
8. Video Games Day
9. National Sugar Cookie Day
10. Don't Step on a Bee Day
11. World Population Day
12. National Pecan Pie Day
13. Day in History: US patent #1 is granted (1836) for locomotive wheels
14. Day in History: First color television broadcast of a sports event (1951)
15. Cow Appreciation Day
16. Toss Away the "Could Haves" and "Should Haves" Day
17. National Peach Ice Cream Day
18. National Caviar Day
19. Day in History: First in-flight movie shown on an airplane (1961)
20. Lollipop Day
21. National Tug-of-War Tournament Day
22. Rat-catchers Day
23. National Vanilla Ice Cream Day
24. Cousins Day
25. Health, Happiness, and Hypnosis Day
26. All or Nothing Day
27. Take Your Houseplant for a Walk Day
28. National Milk Chocolate Day
29. Day in History: The royal wedding of Prince Charles and Lady Diana (1981)
30. National Cheesecake Day
31. Parents Day

August

August is Happiness Happens Month.

1. National Night Out
2. National Ice Cream Sandwich Day
3. National Watermelon Day
4. Twins Day
5. National Mustard Day
6. Friendship Day
7. Professional Speakers Day
8. Happiness Happens Day
9. National Polka Day
10. Lazy Day
11. Presidential Joke Day
12. Elvis Presley Commemoration Day
13. International Left Hander's Day
14. Victory Day
15. National Relaxation Day
16. Day in History: The first issue of *Sports Illustrated* (1954)
17. National Thriftshop Day
18. Bad Poetry Day
19. Potato Day
20. National Radio Day
21. National Spumoni Day
22. Southern Hemisphere Hoodie Hoo Day
23. National Spongecake day
24. Knife Day
25. Kiss-and-Makeup Day
26. Women's Equality Day
27. Petroleum Day
28. World Sauntering Day
29. More Herbs, Less Salt Day
30. National Toasted Marshmallow Day
31. Love Your Lawyer Day

September

September is Healthy Aging Month.

1. Emma M. Nutt Day (first female phone operator, signed on 1878)
2. Day in History: First transatlantic roundtrip flight (1936)
3. Skyscraper Day
4. Newspaper Carrier Appreciation Day
5. Be Late Day
6. Fight Procrastination Day
7. Pardon Day
8. International Literacy Day
9. Teddy Bear Day
10. National Grandparents Day
11. Patriot Day
12. National Pet Memorial Day
13. Fortune Cookie Day

14. National Crème-Filled Donut Day
15. Someday
16. Appreciate Your Wife Day
17. Women's Friendship Day
18. National Play-doh Day
19. National Butterscotch Pudding Day
20. National Punch Day
21. International Day of Peace
22. American Business Women's Day
23. National Hunting and Fishing Day
24. Innergize Day
25. National One-Hit Wonder Day
26. National Good Neighbor Day
27. Women's Health and Fitness Day
28. Ask a Stupid Question Day
29. VFW (Veterans of Foreign Wars) Day
30. Family Health and Fitness Day

October

October is National Breast Cancer Awareness Month.

1. World Vegetarian Day
2. National Custodial Workers Day
3. Day in History: the Mickey Mouse Club premiered on television (1955)
4. National Golf Day
5. National Depression Screening Day
6. Physician Assistants Day
7. International Frugal Fun Day
8. American Tag Day
9. Columbus Day
10. World Mental Health Day
11. Emergency Nurses Day
12. International Moment of Frustration Scream Day
13. World Egg Day
14. National Dessert Day
15. Sunday School Teacher Appreciation Day
16. National Boss's Day
17. Gaudy Day
18. No Beard Day
19. Evaluate Your Life Day
20. Mammography Day
21. Sweetest Day
22. Mother-in-Law Day
23. National Mole Day
24. United Nations Day
25. Sourest Day
26. Mule Day
27. Cranky Co-Workers Day
28. Make a Difference Day
29. Internet Day
31. Halloween
31. National Unicef Day

November

November is National Hospice Month.

1. National Authors Day
2. National Men Make Dinner Day
3. Cliché Day
4. Sadie Hawkins Day
5. Day in History: First post office established in the US in Massachusetts (1639)
6. Saxophone Day
7. National Bittersweet Chocolate with Almonds Day
8. National Parents as Teachers Day
9. Return Day
10. Forget-me-not Day
11. Veterans Day
12. I Need a Patch for That Day
13. World Kindness Day
14. Loosen Up and Lighten Up Day
15. National Educational Support Professionals Day
16. Great American Smokeout
17. Take a Hike Day
18. National Family Volunteer Day
19. Remembrance Day
20. National Adoption Day
21. World Hello Day
22. National Humane Society Anniversary Day
23. Turkey-Free Thanksgiving Day
24. Thanksgiving Day
25. International Day for the Elimination of Violence Against Women
26. Shopping Reminder Day
27. Pins and Needles Day
28. Day in History: the first Polaroid camera is sold
29. Square Dance Day
30. Stay Home Because You're Well Day

December

December is Universal Human Rights Month.

1. National Pie Day
2. Coats for Kids Day
3. International Day of Disabled Persons
4. Extraordinary Work Team Recognition Day
5. National Sacher Torte Day
6. National Gazpacho Day
7. National Cotton Candy Day
8. Day in History: I Love Lucy is first TV show to acknowledge pregnancy (1952)
9. Day of the Horse
10. Human Rights Day
11. International Mountain Day

12. Poinsettia Day
13. Day in History: Dickens' *A Christmas Carol* is published (1843)
14. Day in History: DNA is created in a test tube (1967)
15. Underdog Day
16. National Chocolate-Covered Anything Day
17. Wright Brothers Day
18. International Migrants Day
19. Oatmeal Muffin Day
20. Games Day
21. Winter Solstice
22. Abilities Day
23. Roots Day
24. Christmas Eve
25. Christmas Day
26. National Whiner's Day
27. National Fruitcake Day
28. Card Playing Day
29. No Interruptions Day
30. National Bicarbonate of Soda Day
31. New Year's Eve

APPENDIX VI

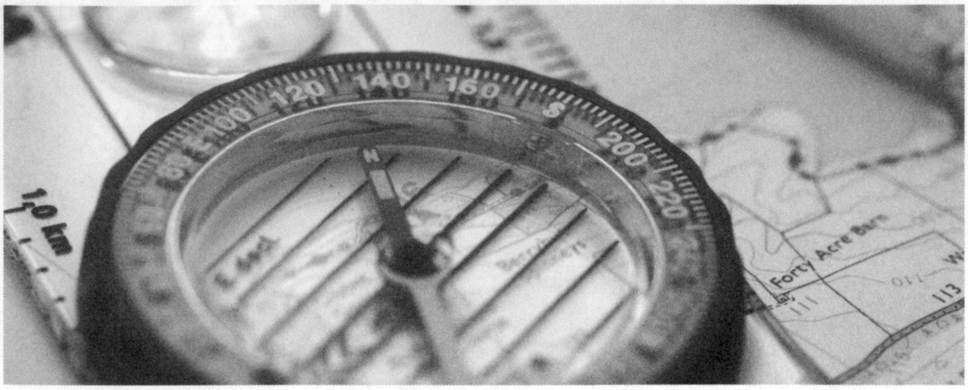

Recommended Books About Marketing

Capellini, Steve. *Massage Therapy Career Guide for Hands-On Success.* 2nd ed. Thomson Delmar Learning. 2006.

Holloway, Colleen. *Success Beyond Work: What Prosperous Massage Therapists Know—Minimum Work, Maximum Profits, and a Sellable Business.* Saramore Publishing Company. 2003.

Levinson, J. *Geurrilla Marketing: Secrets for Making Big Profits from Your Small Business.* 3rd ed. Houghton Mifflin. 1998.

Roseberry, M. *Marketing Massage: From First Job to Dream Practice.* Thomson Delmar Learning. 2006.

Sohnen-Moe, C. *Business Mastery: A Guide for Creating a Fulfilling, Thriving Business and Keeping It Successful.* 3rd ed. Lippincott Williams & Wilkins. 2004.

Stephenson, J. *Entrepreneur Magazine's Ultimate Small Business Marketing Guide: Over 1500 Great Marketing Tricks That Will Drive Your Business Through the Roof.* 2nd ed. Entrepreneur Press. 2006.

Vandepass, Michelle. *Marketing for the Holistic Practitioner.* Conscious Destiny Productions. 2003.

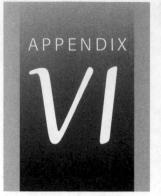

INDEX